# Non-violent Resistance Innovations in Practice

Edited by Elisabeth Heismann, Julia Jude and Elizabeth Day

# Non-violent Resistance Innovations in Practice

## A handbook for anyone working with carers and parents of children and young people who show violent or challenging behaviours



**Published by:**
Pavilion Publishing and Media Ltd
Rayford House
School Road
Hove
East Sussex
BN3 5HX
Tel: 01273 434 943
Fax: 01273 227 308
Email: info@pavpub.com

Published 2019



A catalogue record for this book is available from the British Library.

ISBN: 978-1-912755-08-0



**Editors:** Elisabeth Heismann, Julia Jude and Elizabeth Day
**Cover design:** Emma Dawe, Pavilion Publishing and Media Ltd.
**Page layout and typesetting:** Emma Dawe, Pavilion Publishing and Media Ltd.
**Printing:** Print2Demand Ltd

# Contents

# About the editors

**Dr Elizabeth Day** is a systemic psychotherapist, an artist, a writer, a supervisor and an educator. She established the first NVR group programme in partnership with colleagues in Oxleas NHS Foundation Trust. She and Elisabeth Heismann co-authored the NVR groupwork manual *Non-violent Resistance Programme* published by Pavilion in 2010. Elizabeth Day chose to make the NVR group programme the subject of her doctoral research and was awarded her degree by the University of Bedfordshire in 2015. Elizabeth has worked in schools, residential care, social services and the NHS. Since she retired from full time employment in the NHS she has developed a portfolio career. She teaches and supervises on the Professional Doctorate in Systemic Practice, she is a deputy editor of *Murmurations: Journal of Transformative Systemic Practice*, she has an honorary position as a family therapist in an adult mental health team and she maintains a small private therapy and supervision practice.

**Elisabeth Heismann** is a qualified teacher, systemic therapist, supervisor and trainer with over 10 years of NVR experience. Between 2006 and 2016, together with her colleagues from Health and Social Care, she delivered and led the NVR parent groups within the Oxleas Mental Health Foundation Trust. Elisabeth also developed and ran specialist NVR groups for parents whose children are in gangs or affected by child sexual exploitation for three years in the community. After her retirement from the NHS in 2016, she co-founded the community enterprise company NVR Action and Practice CIC with Dr Julia Jude, offering bespoke NVR training packages for parents and professionals. Elisabeth's special interest is parent participation in NVR. Her current focus is parent mentoring, retention of graduate parents and expansion of the participatory approach in all areas of NVR practice.

**Julia Jude** is a lecturer at London, Goldsmiths University, a visiting lecturer at University of Bedfordshire, a systemic and group psychotherapist, supervisor, researcher, author and co-director of a community project. Her research interests are post-colonial political philosophy, informed by alternative communities of indigenous practice. Over the last few years she has researched the practice of indigenous ideas as a way of providing an alternative therapeutic frame to the contribution of indigenous literature and research within the systemic and social work practice and education.

# Foreword: Finding a way out of the spiral!

**Professor Arist von Schlippe**

It was in 1999 that I met Haim Omer for the first time. Being a trainer in family therapy and systemic therapy in Germany, and also a scientist, I was immediately thrilled by the idea of introducing NVR into the field of counselling and therapy. It is an obvious fit: a communication system that is stuck in struggles for power leads all actors almost unavoidably into a dilemma. They see themselves being forced to choose between only two options, neither of which are very pleasant at all: either escalate the fight or step back and give in.

And both options are usually destructive, as Gregory Bateson has already pointed out. Bateson's research with tribes in Papua New Guinea showed that systems that had not developed a kind of structure to deal with escalation, that had not found rituals for reconciliation, would end up in what he called a 'schismogenetic' process, i.e. a split. This means breaking up the relationship, or, if this is not possible, it means endless circles of fighting, violence, guilt, confusion and rage – in short, the pathways that led to war. In families, this process can be reduced to a simple formula: when a family begins to organise itself around power, when power becomes the organising principle of family communication, then the relationships are jeopardised: power comes in, loving leaves.

This is one of the tragic aspects of power struggles. Bateson had already been very clear in warning of what he called the biggest 'epistemological error' of mankind: to believe in the myth of power. He said that the idea of power corrupts and leads inevitably to disaster. Attempts to establish a satisfying relationship by means of power and violence will always fail, as the dynamic of control will never come to a peaceful end. In families, this means that a relationship, which is already endangered by power struggles, falls even more out of balance, becoming more and more lopsided.

So, instead of trying to win a fight, it would – at least in families – be far better to focus on re-attachment, which of course in an escalatory mind-set is seen as impossible. 'Then he/she might think they have won the fight…' is the usual answer. This creates a vicious circle, in Germany described by the common saying 'the cat bites its own tail'.

Two things are important to highlight here. One is that focusing on repairing relationships is easily associated with 'giving-in', i.e. it will quickly be connected to weakness and defeat by the actors. The other aspect revealed by such an answer is the mindset that fighting can't be stopped by any other means than winning (or losing). No other option is available other than to escalate matters to a point where this final resolution is achieved.

NVR provides a different answer. First, focusing on the relationship doesn't mean becoming weak at all, but uses a different kind of strength: the strength of the anchor is fundamentally different from the strength of the fist. Second, it's the escalation itself that is the problem. So instead of fighting an antagonist and blaming them for problems, NVR fights the escalation itself – if there should be an enemy at all, then it's the communication pattern that has developed.

Trying to solve a relationship issue by exerting power  or using violence is futile and will only serve to aggravate the situation. Conflict systems in escalatory spirals turn into what are called 'highly integrated systems' – and this is not a positive concept at all: in the escalation, the action of one of the partners reduces the options of the other, who then thinks that he cannot act in any way but to give the escalation screw another twist. More and more, the antagonists turn into slaves to this dynamic that they have created together. The self-organising process of escalation has in effect become the problem. And the challenge for counsellors is to turn this negative dynamic into a positive one.

To again relate to Bateson, the conflict system has become a 'context marker' for those involved: whatever the other does or says is framed in a negative way (we know this as the 'hostile attributional error'), so even a constructive attempt by them will be reframed as a negative trick and lead to further escalation. Parental presence, the strength of the anchor, provides a new form of context marker that interrupts this negative communication pattern. The framing must be put in a way that cannot be misunderstood: we as parents are strong, but our strength is not directed against you, our strength is patience and tenacity. And gestures of reconciliation underline the invitation into a different pattern.

NVR thus offers the chance to generate a kind of third way between escalating and giving in. Haim Omer's idea of introducing NVR into counselling has rapidly convinced thousands of professionals across Europe. I know this from Germany where 200,000 copies of the books that Haim and I wrote have been printed in the last 15 years, and this is similar in many other European countries. Professionals are keen to have instruments to contain escalation and stop it from spreading. They know how quickly it can move outside the family and lead to fighting between parents and teachers, teachers and social workers, social workers and parents and so on.

The interventions, and even more the stance of NVR, have the ability to stop these spirals, turning escalating systems back into co-operative ones.

Of course, working in this field is not by any means a piece of cake. On many different levels work has to be done, and practical experiences have to be collected and discussed. This happens in conferences that offer the opportunity to exchange expert knowledge, and this happens in books. One of these books, dear reader, is the one you are now looking at. It is full of information, of operating and hands-on-experiences written by specialists. Some of them belong to the first generation of experts who, in close co-operation with Haim Omer, helped bring NVR to life in so many practical fields. The emerging themes that come up in therapy are described, the intense feelings of helpless parents, their rage and shame that therapists are confronted with, become visible.

You, as a reader, can accompany the authors on the journeys that they went on with their clients, the journeys of change that they initiated and experienced, and you can reflect on the different fields of action – in any of these fields, the basic ideas of NVR have to be adjusted to the respective contexts. Retracing all these stories will help you to find your very own way of applying the basic ideas of non-violence to your particular field of practice. If it is your first encounter, I hope you will be as filled with passion as I was in 1999, and if you are an experienced reader, I wish you a challenging and enriching experience in reading this valuable book.

Witten, Germany
August, 2018

# Non-violent resistance: innovations in practice

## Introduction

This book is made up of chapters that show the myriad ways in which non-violent resistance (NVR) has grown since its original conception as a clinical application by Haim Omer and his team in Tel Aviv (Omer, 2000; 2004; 2010). In understanding how NVR can be used in many contexts, and spring up in very different places, we draw on the idea of rhizomatic connection (Deleuze & Guattari, 1987): 'horizontally linked non-hierarchical forms of social organisation, thought and communication' (Reynolds, 2014, p131). A rhizome, sometimes called a creeping rootstalk, is the stem of a plant that sends out roots and shoots as it spreads. Each of the chapters in this book is rooted in the original NVR ideas but has found a way of expressing itself which is both individual and connected.

When we (Elisabeth, Julia and Elizabeth) thought about writing this introduction, we were struck by the different ways in which clinicians and practitioners relate to NVR as an intervention, and the range of theoretical families to which each belongs. Sometimes the interventions have developed in such an individual way that they look almost like a new entity, but they remain connected under the surface. Each is part of an ever expanding rhizomatic system and remains connected but can break off and grow on its own.

This introduction is divided into three parts. First of all, the three of us set out some of our shared theoretical roots, then we each contribute our own and make connections with the wider field, and finally we introduce the variety of ideas and contexts which awaits you in the book.

For those readers who are relatively new to the concept of NVR, a glossary is included on page 291 to give an introduction to some of these basic ideas and interventions, which will be referred to throughout this book.

# Part 1: shared theoretical roots

We begin the book with the systemic social constructionist theories and ideas which underpin our own NVR practice. We feel it is important for readers to understand the range and complexity of the rhizomatic connections that we have made, because they inform the ways in which we 'do' NVR and are part of our lived practice.

## Narrative and systemic influences

Our therapeutic groupwork programme was developed within the UK's National Health Service (NHS). The three of us were employed as systemic psychotherapists in the same NHS mental health trust where we all worked in the child and adolescent mental health service (CAMHS). The programme was a response to the need to find ways of working with families whose children were presenting with out-of-control and violent behaviours in the face of which the parents felt helpless. The programme is grounded in a systemic approach and uses systemic and narrative methods and techniques such as circular questions, deconstructing episodes, reframing, internalised other interviewing, re-storying, outsider witnessing teams, enactment and sculpting.

Systemic family therapy pays attention to the many stories that exist within families, particularly those untold and unheard stories of strength and resilience (Pearce, 1994; Roberts, 1994; White & Epston, 1990). It values clients as important authors of these new stories and as experts in 'local knowledge' (Geertz, 1983), namely the ways in which their own families work. In the non-violent resistance therapy programme, 'graduate parents' are parents who have successfully completed the programme and are invited to speak about their experiences to new parents and to participate in our future work. This role acknowledges and harnesses their strength and expertise. The power balance is shifted so that parents contribute to one another's learning and insights and to the ongoing development and design of the programme itself.

One of the arts of making the interactions therapeutic is to always be on the lookout for any change, no matter how small, that can then be nurtured and amplified (Tomm *et al*, 2014). Small changes are noticed, attention is drawn to them, they are asked about in detail, and then developed. It is like looking for the tiny end of a thread, which can be teased out and developed into a story (White, 1991; Roberts, 1994), which can then be thickened and enriched (Geertz, 1973). When families have a repertoire of thin and problem-saturated accounts of their lives (Lang & McAdam, 1995), therapists work to create fuller stories.

Storytelling is a standard systemic narrative technique. In NVR, parents begin to develop the skill to use it themselves and, in an NVR group setting, enthusiastically start doing it for one another. This is an example of second-order learning (Schön, 1983). When we focus on moments of revelation (also called a light-bulb or 'ah ha!' moments), we notice that more of them happen and that parents are noticing them too. This amplifies the effect of these moments; the act of noticing creates more moments, or a greater sensitivity to them, which in turn is mirrored in an enhanced sensitivity in the parents to their own and others' experiences.

Vygotsky (1978) describes this interesting aspect of collaborative learning as the 'zone of proximal development' (ZPD). When people learn together, the space (zone) becomes one in which learning is optimised and extended. Vygotsky also highlights the importance in this process of the 'More Knowledgeable Other' (MKO): the parent who leads the way by being able to describe their own experience for others, who can then visualise and learn from it. Vygotsky highlights the role that helpers play in learning – that people learn more quickly and achieve more if someone else is there with them, providing guidance and encouragement. Graduate parents perform this role in our group programme. Parents whose relationships have already started to improve are able to perform this role for those who are still struggling – they embody hope for the rest of the group. Each time a parent tells a story of struggle and movement, they enrich the story of the group as a place where change happens.

## Specific influences

**Social constructionism** (Burr, 1995; Gergen, 2001; 2009; McNamee & Gergen, 1992; Tomm *et al*, 2014). We believe that meaning is constructed between people in conversation and interaction.

**The Milan School** (Boscolo *et al*, 1987; Cecchin, 1987; Cecchin *et al*, 1992) introduced the concepts of circular questioning, curiosity, inviting different perspectives, noticing differences and prejudices, and irreverence; and some of the strategies for evoking those differences: techniques like prescriptions and sculpting.

**Minuchin** (1974) demonstrated the power of using oneself as an actor in the session: moving people about, challenging unhelpful alliances, using his position as an older and more respected clinician to provoke and perturb the system.

**Narrative Therapy** (White & Epston, 1990) introduced practices like storytelling, re-storying, witnessing and insider witnessing teams. This informs the ways in which we seek out stories, look for exceptions and unique outcomes, and ask outsiders who have been in the same situation to come in and share their stories.

 

**Psychodrama** (Moreno, 1987) developed our ideas about sculpting, rehearsal and performance. It is used in the ways in which we encourage participants to try speaking out loud, reading out their announcements, imagining how it feels to hear the announcement from a different position. Augusto Boal (1979) developed his 'Theatre of the Oppressed' in the 1970s in Brazil, and later in Europe, as an instrument for personal and social change.

**The Co-ordinated Management of Meaning** (CMM) (Cronen *et al*, 1982; Pearce, 1989; 1994; 2007; Pearce & Pearce, 1998; Oliver, 1996) gave us a theoretical framework for exploring storytelling, beliefs, contextual and implicative forces, stories from communities and families, and ideas about deconstructing episodes and exploring meanings. We work to unpick strange loops in parent-child interactions and expose the beliefs that have held them in place.

**Reflecting teams** (Andersen, 1987) provides the foundation for much of the way in which we observe and reflect in front of group members, reframing action, opening up new possibilities, and giving meaning to how to go on.

**Embodiment** (Shotter, 2010; 2012; 2016) writings emphasise the importance of becoming aware how emotion is held physically in the body. The use of relaxation and mindfulness helps participants become more attuned to their emotions, allowing them to learn to connect and act from a calmer and more thoughtful place.

**Open dialogue** (Seikkula & Olson, 2003; Seikkula & Trimble, 2005; Rober, 2005) dialogical approaches and conversations on the margins of meaning-making have been very useful to us. There is a dialogical recursive effect when stories are co-constructed in a group. In their paper *Healing elements of therapeutic conversation: dialogue as an embodiment of love*, Seikkula and Trimble (2005) identify particular therapeutic elements that facilitate healing.

> *'Certain experiences have come to mark for us turning points in the healing process. They include strong collective feelings of sharing and belonging together; emerging expressions of trust; embodied expressions of emotion; feelings of relief of tension experienced as physical relaxation; and, perhaps surprisingly, ourselves becoming involved in strong emotions and evidencing love.'*

Here, Seikkula and Trimble are describing the qualities that make the open dialogue approach (Seikkula & Olson, 2003) work so well, but their description also fits the NVR therapy programme.

In the preface to their book *Systemic Therapy as Transformative Practice*, Simon and McCarthy write, '*We are using the word "systemic" to portray fluidly responsive practices with an ethical preoccupation about what makes a difference, for whom and how*' (McCarthy & Simon, 2016, pxiv). This neatly describes the ethical basis upon which we act when delivering NVR as a systemic therapeutic groupwork practice.

# Part 2: The people and ideas that influenced us

## Elisabeth

I was born in Germany after the war, the youngest of three. My oldest brother had physical, behavioural and emotional disabilities, which I experienced with some ambivalence of love, shame and embarrassment, growing up in an era that had to come to terms with the murder of Jews, gay people, people from the travelling communities, as well as 5,000 people with mental health problems (called 'handicapped') under the Nazi regime.

Belonging to the generation of 1968 that rebelled against any form of repression and social injustice and re-armament, I supported worldwide movements against oppression, colonialism, apartheid and social injustices. This brought me in contact with Latin American liberation theology and education, which was based on the understanding that peace cannot be attained without the complete liberation of the people. In 1977, I was very moved by the news of a small farming community on the island of Solentiname in Nicaragua. Together with the liberation priest and poet Ernesto Cardenal, the farmers occupied a barrack to protest against the Nicaraguan dictator Samoza, resulting in the complete destruction of their church and village.

When, in 2015, I visited the small chapel in Solentiname they had rebuilt, and I experienced the small rural community that Ernesto Cardenal had given such a powerful voice in his book *The Gospel in Solentiname* (Cardenal, 1976), I felt very emotional and privileged. I was a keen supporter of Allende's socialist government in Chile in the early 70s, which found its brutal end with the bombing of the government palace, 'The Moneda', on 11th September 1973. On a recent visit to Chile in 2017, I stood at the graves of the singer-songwriters Violetta Parra, Víctor Jara and of President Salvador Allende and saw the houses of the poet Pablo Neruda, feeling deeply moved and still very connected to the years of Allende.

All these Latin-American priests, politicians, educators, poets and musicians and the communities that they had influenced, were convinced of the need for revolutionary changes in their countries and refused to be intimidated by the power of dictators or traditional hierarchies, but followed their conscience and faith instead, often with the consequence of death, exile and imprisonment.

Between 1985 and 1988 I lived in Zimbabwe as I wanted to experience first-hand the building of a country post colonialism. At this time I came across the writings of Frantz Fanon about the influence of colonialism and racism on black and white identities (Fanon 2001; 2017). I also got involved in the indigenous approach to medicine and healing, when, for about one year, I worked with a healer, midwife and spiritual medium. I collected herbal medicines with her, as well as observing her putting herself into trance and treating people.

When living in Zimbabwe, I was first introduced to systemic thinking and ways of working, when, in 1987, we formed the first family therapy team in Harare of mainly non-therapeutically trained professionals (including social workers and a policeman). Together we saw large family systems with sometimes 15 or more adult members.

When moving to the UK in 1988, where I studied systemic therapy, I incorporated these less orthodox approaches to therapy and family work. I co-founded Upper Street Multi-Cultural Counselling Centre in 1991, a charity with a team of volunteer therapists.

Since the early 80s I have been using 'loving kindness' (Salzberg, 2002; Goldstein 2003), which is a Tibetan form of meditation practice, that – according to tradition – was taught by the Buddha to help monks conquer their fear. This practice has not only been helpful in my own life but has also supported people's transformation journey in NVR. I have learned that social and personal liberation, transformation and change cannot be prescribed or dictated, but can only happen when they are based on acceptance, perseverance, the concept of interconnectedness, compassion, love, forgiveness and participation.

I am deeply committed to a continuous development of NVR practices and theories, making them more accessible, transparent, participatory and adaptable to the lives and relationships of those in the community who are suffering from the de-humanising effects of isolation, injustice, oppression and racism on their relationships.

## Julia

In 1956, Pierre Bourdieu and Jean Claude Passeron suggested that 'academic ideas, knowledge and ways of knowing is dead, wooden and lifeless knowledge'.

They suggested that the way in which knowledge is articulated is no-one's mother tongue, which implies that what counts as knowledge is socially constructed and not naturally inherited by the individuals, groups or communities.

The term 'dead language' resonates with me. My professional habits of doing research and practice had erased memories of my ancestral tradition of doing practice, leaving me to rehearse and put in place predicted knowledge and ideas that were not my own. What was removed was the appreciation of my culturally inherited context and the ordinary ways in which my ancestors gave meaning to life. What was removed was the vibrancy of hearing stories of lived experiences that gave meaning to my life.

So, when I came across Haim Omer's work, I found myself drawn to his ideas and practice. Why? Instead of citing the usual suspects in the scholarly and academic fields, Omer stepped out from the habitual ways of presenting his ideas by choosing to celebrate the works of Gandhi, Martin Luther King and Rosa Parks. Political activists and people of colour who spoke out against issues of social injustice. This was a critical moment for me. As the NVR approach touched on my historical and ancestral history of oppression, social injustice and discrimination, it reinforced the need for change in the ways that we validate knowledge, but more importantly, emphasised ways in which we make sense of our relationship through 'praxis': 'embodied' experiences in our everyday action and responses. NVR's tradition in political activisms leads me to interrogate my relationship with the type of knowledge that I wanted to engage with and nurture. It helped me to create opportunities for rethinking how to unlearn the usual practice of establishing hierarchal structures that placed traditional scholarly knowledge at the helm.

This required a posture of critical awareness: of how I changed where I go to gather knowledge that would enable me to find ways of dialoguing and performing stories that offered relational accounts of our relationship with others.

Paying attention to the voices of others enabled alternative dialogue, learning and creativity to emerge. The rhizomatic connection was pivotal in the process of expanding my relationship with knowledge which lent itself to the continuity of rethinking, of always inviting alternative learning and knowledge that would reflect inclusivity of ideas and practices. This required a decolonising approach to how we interact with knowledge, that allows us to rethink our practice, ideas and discourses.

This process led to the inclusion of the works of indigenous scholars, whose ideas sit outside traditional Western academic spheres. In doing so, we were keen to put forward scholarly voices that offer an alternative view as one way of generating creative practices, learning and development. By including alternative knowledge, we wanted to expand on where our knowledge would take us and the new practice that could be afforded to us.

## Elizabeth

I came to NVR with a passion for community and user involvement. The thread that runs through my life is one of working with marginalised people and helping them find a voice: lesbian mothers whose children had been removed by the courts; women on bail awaiting trial; young people living in children's homes; gay and bisexual men with HIV; drug users; African families affected by HIV; children and young people with mental health problems; lesbian, gay, bisexual and trans (LGBT+) users of mental health services; people living with cancer.

The role of graduate parents as collaborators in the development of NVR as a group intervention emerged naturally and organically. For example, the self-announcement (Day & Heismann, 2010) came about when a group of mothers were struggling to write an announcement. They spoke about things from the past that they felt had contributed to their current situation (domestic violence, alcohol and drug use), feeling that they somehow deserved what was happening at home. One of the mothers said, '*You know some people aren't ready to write an announcement. We need to forgive ourselves first, to believe that we can be good mothers, whatever has happened in the past, and we deserve to expect things to be better*'. In this way we co-constructed the idea of the self-announcement which has become one of the most powerful moments in the process.

The way in which facilitators, parents and carers perform (Denzin, 2006) the principles of NVR (de-escalation, reconciliation and love) means that those transformations are communicated in the group at a level which is profound in its effect.

### To sum it up...

All these above influences and practices have now found a new and natural home in our approach to NVR. Love may not be enough (Crittenden, 2008; Ingamells & Epston, 2014), but it is central to the posture that we need to adopt and model.

# Part 3: what the book contains

We believe that the roots of NVR are to be found among those individuals, like Gandhi or Martin Luther King, who believed in making a better and fairer world, who acted outside the usual frame and were positioned at the forefront of their movements. Connection, participation, collaboration, reflecting-on and reflecting-in practice are all key elements of this approach. We have therefore decided to include the voices of parents, practitioners and first-time writers on the same stage as established authors, indigenous scholars and academics. Where people are writing in English, and it is not their first language, we have tried to preserve some of the flavour of their voice, because doing so gives voice also to their community; this is a reflexive and performative process. We hope it will encourage those who have not yet told their stories to feel that they have something to offer.

We have grouped the chapters into five sections: emerging themes, working for a better future, working with difference, working with groups, and working in and with schools. We asked authors to include examples from practice to illustrate their writing.

## Part 1: Emerging themes

These first seven chapters describe developments in NVR and in New Authority (Omer, 2010) thinking and practice.

Uri Weinblatt explores the impact of shame on children, adolescents and parents. He deconstructs episodes and shows in detail how shame, hurt and blame are connected and can escalate situations.

Haim Omer & Naama Gershy write about the value of fathers in child development and how to engage them in situations where there is parental conflict or separation, or when fathers are unused to participating actively in childcare. They offer practical suggestions for managing fathers' reluctance to become involved and encouraging collaboration between parents.

Julia Jude and Veronica Rivera-Gould develop this theme in their chapter. They set the literature about fathers within a wider framework and critique the prevalence of Eurocentric approaches to making meaning of gendered parenting roles. They bring in the voices of fathers who were interviewed about their experiences of participating in NVR groups, and address changing relationships, changing engagement and perceptions of fathering in NVR.

Peter Jakob examines what happens between parents, caregivers and children when trauma blunts responses. He describes how parents and caregivers can rekindle a 'caring dialogue' in order to carry on, and enable the child to accept their overtures of care.

Julia Jude sets out a theoretical framework within which she explores NVR as a safeguarding intervention with parents. She draws on the literature about how we learn and connects this to the benefits of coaching. Sarah Blyth joins the conversation and describes how NVR empowered her to take a different position with her son who was involved in gang-related activities. Sarah speaks about the importance for parents of being encouraged to practise their NVR skills in order to move forward.

Linda Cakebread describes how she has used NVR in adult mental health services in London. She describes situations where parents of adult children were finding it hard to resist their children's demands. This is a practical application of NVR by someone who has in the past been in the situation of a parent needing help herself.

Frank Van Holen & Johann Vanderfaeille carry out a critical review of NVR and New Authority through a review of the literature. They compare and contrast the two approaches and explore who uses each intervention, in which contexts and with what problematic behaviours. The effectiveness of NVR as an intervention is reviewed through the literature.

## Part 2: Working for a better future

We have chosen the three chapters in this section because they stand out for their passion for bringing about change at a macro level.

Ziv Gilad has called his chapter 'Building trust and co-operation between Israeli Police and Israeli-Arab Citizens'. Ziv describes a pilot study comparing the behaviour of two groups of recently qualified police officers in a simulated conflict situation; one had received training in constructive struggle and the other (the control group) had not. This interesting study has implications for the training of police in any country where there is a climate of high conflict.

Zoe McLeod and Gill Westwood show how their NVR approach to young people who find themselves before the courts is situated within a much wider commitment to improving the lives of disadvantaged families in their inner-city area.

Elisabeth Heismann, Julie Pierzchniak and Jane Prescott reflect on the experience of developing and running specialist NVR groups for parents whose children are gang members, or affected by gangs, and those exposed to child sexual exploitation. They describe how the NVR approach enables them to work with and alongside families taken hostage by a culture of poverty, deprivation and divided loyalties.

## Part 3: Working with difference

Julia Jude argues for a radical rethink of the discourses around parenting for Black, Asian and Minority Ethnic families and those agencies who work with them. She suggests that NVR principles are well placed to be integrated with post-colonial thinking.

Emma Fayter writes about the experience of running NVR groupwork programmes in culturally diverse neighbourhoods. She describes tailoring NVR to meet the particular cultural needs of the local Bangladeshi community.

Gilda Flores A describes developing and delivering NVR programmes for Latin American families in London. Many Latin Americans do not access health and social care, are isolated, work anti-social hours and are far away from their traditional networks of support. Gilda shows how communities of parents can be created and support networks can evolve through a culturally specific NVR programme in Spanish.

Carole Payne contributes an individual case study which describes her clinical work with a mixed heritage family in southern England.

## Part 4: Working with groups

Elizabeth Day locates NVR groups within the wider history of groupwork and the context of parenting programmes.

In Chapter 16, Elisabeth Heismann explains the theoretical and political underpinnings of the participatory approach. This is a rich description of the ideas and literature which inform the participation of graduate parents in the NVR programmes.

This is followed by a fascinating free-flowing conversation about the value of parent participation by the people who developed it and the parents who have taken it forward and made it their own.

Pete Brown sets out an array of practical advice for parents within the NVR and wider literature. He introduces specific phrases that enable parents to begin the process of reconnecting with their children. Pete also describes how parents can protect themselves from hurt in order to remain calm in their journey towards better relationships.

 

## Part 5: Working in and with schools

Delegates who attended the 2017 NVR UK conference were asked what topics they wanted covered in future training. Work in schools was the area which received the most votes.

Dorota Rospierska and Kyla Evans describe their NVR work within school communities in south east London, giving a detailed account of developing and nurturing NVR in schools and locating their practice within the wider systemic framework.

Idan Amiel and Tal Maimon describe their ground-breaking programme in schools. They use NVR principles to empower teachers and create support networks to reduce problematic behaviour among students. They reach out to parents and enable them to participate in school interventions.

# Final reflections

The process of writing this introduction has been fascinating. We have each contributed to the content and to the overall shape.

Frank and Johann point out in their chapter that, in some parts of the world, New Authority has become the preferred theoretical concept, but we have chosen to remain faithful to NVR. In our experience of working with parents we are drawn to the NVR approach because it is a reflexive, fluid and systemic way of working with relationships. NVR also has strong historical connections with universal social struggle and political action across the globe.

Shame comes through as a recurrent theme in many of the papers. There is a recognition that fathers have often been ignored and side-lined in parenting interventions. Julia Jude, Naama Gershy and Haim Omer describe how fathers can be included and encouraged and parents describe how important this is for successful co-parenting, and to redress dominant discourses around parenting.

We need to think outside the box in understanding how parents from different backgrounds have developed their parenting strategies and how those have been affected by oppression: racism, sexism, poverty and homophobia. In addition, we should think creatively about how NVR might be applied in other settings. Ziv Gilad, Linda Cakebread and Zoe McLeod and Gill Westwood give examples of how this is already happening. People are also developing NVR in management settings to work with teams in conflict.

 

We believe that the current emphasis on outcome-based research methods cannot do justice to the transformative effects of NVR as a therapeutic intervention. Action research, also known as action participatory research (McNiff & Whitehead, 2005), has a good fit with evolving practices. Here we would also like to draw attention to Elizabeth Day's doctoral research (2014) in which she developed Rich Portraiture. This is a new practitioner-research method that is a direct response to the complexity of the research task of better understanding why NVR groups are so successful.

The assemblage of chapters raises questions about the different ways in which we might understand and apply NVR in aspects of our day-to-day relationships. What comes through is the real potential for new and innovative practice to emerge rhizomatically by remaining open to and curious about new ways of thinking and doing; creating alternative ways of reforming and disrupting practice.

## References

Andersen T (1987) The Reflective team: dialogue and meta-dialogue in clinical work. *Family Process* **26** pp415–427.

Bateson G (1973) *Steps to an Ecology of Mind*. London: Paladin.

Bateson G (1979) *Mind and Nature*. New York: Dutton.

Boal A (1979) *Theater of the Oppressed*. Pluto Press.

Bourdieu P & Passeron J (1956) *Reproduction in Education, Society and Culture*.

Boscolo L, Cecchin G, Hoffman L & Penn P (1987) *Milan Systemic Family Therapy Conversations in Theory and Practice*. New York: Basic Books.

Burr V (1995) *An Introduction to Social Constructionism*. London: Routledge.

Cardenal E (2007) *The Gospel in Solentiname* (translated by Donald D Walsh). New York: Orbis Books.

Cecchin G (1987) Hypothesising, circularity and neutrality revisited: an invitation to curiosity. *Family Process* **26** pp405–413.

Cecchin G, Lane G & Ray WA (1992) *Irreverence: A strategy for therapists' Survival*. London: Karnac Books.

Crittenden PM (2008) *Raising Parents*. Cullompton: Willan Publishing.

Cronen VE, Johnson KM & Lannamann JW (1982) Paradoxes, double binds, and reflexive loops: an alternative theoretical perspective. *Family Process* **21** (1) 91–112.

Day EM (2014) *A Rich Portrait of the Non-violent Resistance Multi-parent Therapeutic Group Programme*. Unpublished Doctoral Thesis. Available from the University of Bedfordshire Repository.

Day EM & Heismann E (2010) *Non-violent Resistance Programme*. Hove: Pavilion Publishing.

Deleuze G & Guattari F (1987) *A Thousand Plateaus: Capitalism and schizophrenia*. London: Athlone Press.

Denzin NK (2006) 'The politics and ethics of performance pedagogy: Toward a pedagogy of hope'. In: DS Madison & J Hamera (Eds) *The Sage Handbook of Performance Studies*. Thousand Oaks, CA: Sage.

Fanon F (2001) *The Wretched of the Earth*. (translated by Constance Farrington), Penguin Books.

Fanon F (2017) *Black Skin, White Masks* (translated by Charles Lam Markmann). Pluto Press.

Geertz C (1973) *The Interpretation of Cultures: Selected essays*. New York: Basic Books.

Geertz C (1983) *Local Knowledge*. New York: Basic Books.

Gergen KJ (2001) *Social Construction in Context*. London: Sage.

Gergen KJ (2009) *An Invitation to Social Constructionism*. Second Edition. London: Sage.

Goldstein J (2003) *Insight Meditation: The practice of freedom*. Boston and London: Shambala.

Ingamells K & Epston D (2014) Love is not all you need: a revolutionary approach to parental abuse. *Australian and New Zealand Journal of Family Therapy* **35** 364-382.

Lang P & McAdam E (1995) Referrals, referrers and the system of concern. *Human Systems* **6** pp71–103.

McCarthy I & Simon G (Eds) (2016) *Systemic Therapy as Transformative Practice*. Farnhill: Everything is Connected Press.

McNamee S & Gergen KJ (Eds) (1992) *Therapy as Social Construction*. London: Sage.

McNiff J & Whitehead J (2005) *All You Need to Know About Action Research*. London: Sage.

Minuchin S (1974) *Families and Family Therapy*. Cambridge: Harvard University Press.

Moreno JL (1987) *The Essential Moreno*. New York: Springer.

Oliver C (1996) Systemic eloquence. *Human Systems* **7** 247–264.

Omer H (2000) *Parental Presence*. Phoenix: Zeig Tucker & Co Inc.

Omer H (2004) *Non-violent Resistance*. Cambridge: Cambridge University Press.

Omer H (2010) *The New Authority*. Cambridge: Cambridge University Press.

Pearce WB (1989) *Communication and the Human Condition*. Carbondale and Edwardsville: Southern Illinois University Press.

Pearce WB (1994) *Interpersonal Communication: Making Social Worlds*. New York: HarperCollins.

Pearce WB (2007) *Making Social Worlds*. Oxford: Blackwell Publishing.

Pearce WB & Pearce KA (1998) Transcendent storytelling: abilities for systemic practitioners and their clients. *Human Systems* **9** pp167–185.

Reynolds V (2014) 'A Solidarity Approach: The rhizome and messy inquiry'. In: G Simon and A Chard (Eds) *Systemic Inquiry*. Farnhill: Everything is Connected Press.

Rober P (2005) The therapist's self in dialogical family therapy: some ideas about not-knowing and the therapist's inner conversation. *Family Process* **44** (4) 477–95.

Roberts J (1994) *Tales and Transformations*. London: Norton Books.

Salzberg S (2002) *Loving Kindness: The revolutionary art of happiness*. Boston and London: Shambala.

Schön DA (1983) *The Reflective Practitioner: How professionals think in action*. London: Temple Smith.

Seikkula J & Olson ME (2003) The open dialogue approach to acute psychosis: its poetics and micropolitics. *Family Process* **42** (3) pp403–418.

Seikkula J & Trimble D (2005) Healing elements of therapeutic conversation: dialogue as an embodiment of love. *Family Process* **44** (4) pp461–475.

 

Shotter J (2010) *Social Construction on the Edge: Withness-thinking and embodiment.* Taos Institute Publications.

Shotter J (2012) More than Cool Reason: 'Withness-thinking' or 'systemic thinking' and 'thinking about systems'. *International Journal of Collaborative Practices* **3** (1) pp1–13.

Shotter J (2016) *Speaking, Actually: Towards a new 'fluid' common-sense understanding of relational becomings.* Farnhill: Everything is Connected Press.

Strong T & Tomm K (2007) Family Therapy as Re-Coordinating and Moving on Together. *Journal of Systemic Therapies* **26** (2) pp42–54.

Tomm K, St George S, Wulff D & Strong T (2014) *Patterns in Interpersonal Interactions.* London and New York: Routledge.

Vygotsky LS (1978) *Mind in Society: The development of higher psychological processes.* Cambridge, MA: Harvard University Press.

White M (1991) *Re-Authoring Lives: Interviews and essays.* Adelaide: Dulwich Centre Publications.

White M & Epston D (1990) *Narrative Means to Therapeutic Ends.* London: Norton.

 

# Part 1: Emerging themes

# Chapter 1: Regulating shame in NVR

**Uri Weinblatt**

## Introduction

Shame is the emotion most connected with issues of power and hierarchy in the family, and is often the driving force behind power struggles and relationship impasses. When unregulated, shame can make both parents and children feel belittled, humiliated and unappreciated. This chapter demonstrates how NVR interventions can regulate the shame of adolescents and their parents. Specific interventions for regulating states of shamefulness and shamelessness are described.

Shame is a key emotion in the development, maintenance and resolution of interpersonal power struggles and conflict. When shame intensifies, family members often perceive themselves to be in a powerless and subordinate position. Take for example a basic interaction in which a parent demands something from the child. The demand evokes in the child shame, which derives from being in an inferior position. If the child is not compliant with the parental demand ('I am not going to clean my room, you clean it!), it is now the parent who is in an inferior position and who needs to deal with his or her shame. The ability of both child and parent to regulate their shame determines the quality of the relationship they have with one another.

Shame is related to the management of power in relationships and is described as the emotion one feels when one experiences being belittled, inadequate and/or disrespected (Greenberg & Goldman, 2008). This is exactly how parents and children feel when engaged in ongoing intense conflicts. For both sides, these escalating conflicts result in feeling the shame of being disrespected and underappreciated. As shame rises, the rigidity of opinions and mutual power-oriented behaviours on both sides increase. This leaves the system in shame-rage escalation loops, which are hard to escape (Scheff, 1997).

## The effects of shame on family members

When shame is unregulated, attacking the other, withdrawing (Nathanson, 1992) and striving for power become common behaviours between family members. Of these, attacking the other is the most predominant reaction in intense family conflict. In attacking the other, the shamed person feels hurt and inferior, which in turn leads to a sense of being legitimised and even morally obligated to hurt back. In these situations, the person is trying to transfer shame from themselves to others by criticising, blaming, ridiculing, putting down and communicating hateful comments (Kaufman, 1996).

In situations of ongoing family conflict, it is common for parents to experience intense shame. Some of these parents react to their higher levels of shame by losing control and harshly punishing the child, and others by avoidance and giving-in. The weaker and more uninfluential the parent feels, the more the risk of attacking, withdrawing or a combination of the two increases.

When family members experience shame for too long or too intensely, they may try to avoid or eliminate any situation that might arouse the feeling again. In fact, many escalations in family conflicts are caused by the efforts of one party or the other (or both) to stop behaving in ways which are shaming for the other. As a result, any shame-provoking interaction (any demand from another person, any remark, critique, comment or suggestion) can lead to conflict (Gilligan, 2001), or to someone leaving the situation and trying to avoid it altogether.

This process can lead to continual disruptions in relationships and to an inability to communicate authentically. Ultimately, it can lead to the breakdown of dialogue, and turns verbal communication efforts into frustrating and dangerous encounters. In such situations, family members feel they must walk on eggshells, knowing very well that talking freely can lead to intense escalations. It is exactly in these situations that collaborative/communication oriented relational gestures reach their limit.

When shame exceeds a certain threshold, the person's ability to collaborate with others is compromised. For children, intense shame can lead to temper tantrums, noncompliance and a myriad of avoidant behaviours. For adolescents who experience high levels of shame, aggression, self-cutting, drug abuse, refusal to attend school and other dysfunctional behaviours are common behaviours. These teens also persistently refuse to admit to having a problem and refuse to accept help. This attitude often leaves their parents, teachers and therapists in states of helplessness, anger and anxiety because they don't know how to move the child forward when the main path towards progress – verbal communication – is often unavailable.

 

This chapter focuses on how NVR can help such teens regulate their shame. I start by describing one major aspect in regulating shame – the need to regulate situations where it is experienced too strongly (states of shamefulness) and situations in which it is absent (shamelessness). I then present relevant NVR interventions related to regulating both states, and clarify how these interventions can help adolescents reduce their shame (in shameful states) or re-integrate it (in shameless states). While the focus of the chapter is mainly on adolescents, the parents, who are the initiators of the shame regulation interventions, do not remain unaffected – while implementing the interventions, they become more efficient in regulating their own shame.

## The fundamentals of regulating intense shame

Since most teens who experience intense shame refuse to enter therapy (or, when they do, they fail to make it meaningful), the process of change is usually led by the parents (and/or school personnel). The regulation process is tricky because it demands two opposing actions (Weinblatt, 2016):

- Reducing the adolescent's shame when it is experienced too painfully (in states of shamefulness).
- Reintegrating/exposing shame when it is absent (in states of shamelessness).

One of the key problems in addressing intense shame states is that they do not look like shame in the way that we might expect to see it, and it is sometimes hard to recognise as a result. The physical displays of shame: covering the face, lowering the eyes and blushing, are all absent. Instead, we see behaviours we associate with rage or apathy – acting out, loss of control and rage. If we can recognise that it is in fact intense shame we are dealing with, rather than anger or apathy, we can overcome it by reconnecting with the child, even if they forbid and oppose it. The main interventions used in NVR to accomplish this are 'Reconciliation Gestures'.

Shamelessness, on the other hand, is the outcome of an effort by an adolescent to stop caring, and is experienced mostly as apathy, disconnection and withdrawal. It is a reaction to the experience of intense pain and leads to varying degrees of disassociation (De Young, 2015). Through this process the person becomes disconnected from shame. When shame therefore becomes unfelt and absent, the goal is to integrate it back into the teen's life.

Since the ability to tolerate shame is built up by experiencing it at manageable levels, NVR interventions induce shame in ways that allow the child to master it. The exposure to shame is never welcomed by the teen and evokes intense reactions. The two main interventions that assist in achieving these goals are the 'Sit-in' and 'Public Opinion' interventions.

When shame is experienced at moderate levels the adolescent can slowly ease the pain in relatively constructive ways (through dialogue, time-limited withdrawal or non-harmful distractions).

When shame is experienced at moderate levels, the adolescent can slowly ease the pain in relatively constructive ways (through dialogue, time-limited withdrawal or non-harmful distractions). In situations of intense shame, the adolescent shifts intermittently between shamefulness and shamelessness. The intensely shameful reaction creates debilitating emotional pain which can often only be dealt with by distancing, disconnecting and dissociating from it, or simply by becoming shameless. This enables the child to transcend his vulnerability and to feel strong again but at a heavy price – it does not allow him or her to take responsibility for their behaviour, admit their faults, apologise, or to try to repair the damage they have inflicted on others – behaviours which lead to re-connection with others. Without this connection the teen remains alone – a state which leaves them vulnerable to experiencing further shame.

## NVR interventions for states of shamefulness

When adolescents or children experience intense shame, their lives are often marked by many failures. Whether the failures are interpersonal, academic, or in any other domain of life, they often lead parents to suggest what they think are helpful corrections and explanations, and deliver 'educational' lectures. The adolescent on the other hand, often experiences this as criticism, disapproval and blame. Seemingly 'neutral' requests or comments such as, 'Please wash the dishes', 'clean your room', and 'if you continue to talk to your friends like that, they won't be your friends,' can ignite a strong shame reaction.

The first step in reducing an adolescent's shame is for the parents to make a conscious decision to reduce their use of comments that might sound critical. Using the 'three baskets' intervention, parents are coached to refrain from mentioning failures – not cleaning after himself, not keeping a promise, leaving dirty plates around etc. At the same time, parents are also coached to create interpersonal bridges that do not involve evaluation, and which make it less likely that shame will be triggered. For example, they are encouraged to make statements such as: 'I'm thinking about you'; 'I love you' or 'I'm sorry that we had a fight yesterday'. Statements such as these create connections with the child and lower their sense of shame. Moreover, short, supportive sentences of this kind have a preventive function – by providing the adolescent with on-going information as to what is going through the parent's mind, it counters the tendency of shamed adolescents to reach false conclusions by incorrectly 'mind reading' their parents' intentions.

Another type of NVR intervention is 'Reconciliation Gestures', which are highly effective in reducing shame. They include statements expressing respect for the child, suggestions of shared activities, apologies and symbolic gifts.

A parents' reconciliation gestures are unilateral initiatives that are not conditional on the child's positive behaviours. As such they have the potential to evoke corrective emotional experiences for the teen. For example, after lashing out at his parents a teenage boy may well expect to be attacked by the parents in return, and yet instead he receives a positive and forgiving reaction. This unexpected and supportive reaction can be very effective at countering the boy's shameful cognitions ('I am unlovable') and replace them with shame-regulated thoughts ('I have value, my parents care about me').

## NVR interventions for states of shamelessness

Intense shame leads ultimately to states of shamelessness, in which the person essentially disconnects from experiencing shame. This significantly jeopardises their ability to feel empathy (Tangney & Dearing, 2002; Tangney *et al*, 2007), and as a result also reduces their ability to communicate effectively. As the person's capacity to co-operate deteriorates, the relational bridge that connects them to others breaks down, leaving them alone and humiliated. An inability to experience shame can be extremely destructive and can lead either to antisocial or avoidant behaviours. An effective shame regulation model must therefore assist the adolescent to integrate shame back into his or her life, and to re-connect with their sense of shame. In NVR the two main interventions for doing so are the 'Sit-in' and the 'Public Opinion' interventions.

In the sit-in intervention (Omer, 2001), the adolescent is exposed to shame by the parents while being helped to regulate it. The parents evoke shame by:

- Entering and staying in the adolescent's room. This creates a discontinuation of a pleasurable activity for him or her. Tomkins (1963) has suggested that it is exactly these types of activating behaviours that lead to the shame response.
- Focusing on a behaviour that the adolescent feels ashamed of. Whether it is aggressive behaviour, school failures, computer addiction, eating disorders, self-inflicted injury, lack of safe sexual boundaries, cyber bullying or drug

use, the parents bring up an issue in the adolescent's life that feels to him/her like a failure.

- Staying in the child's room without his permission. As such, the parents are not only challenging the teen's sense of autonomy but are renegotiating the boundaries of what is private. This intrusion evokes shame because the adolescent feels that what had previously been considered private has now been turned into a public domain.

After shame has been triggered, the parents' de-escalation actions (such as physically being in a lower position, maintaining self-control, respectful silence and a lack of threatening and aggressive behaviours) reduce the level of shame. As a result the child gets the chance to both experience the emotion and the process of decreasing it. This unique experience leads to positive outcomes (or shame regulation indicators) for both the adolescent and their parents. These include:

- The adolescent can tolerate the state of 'having a problem' and 'needing help'. Issues which were considered taboo can be discussed.
- The adolescent permits his parents to 'see' him and he learns to manage the feeling of being exposed.
- The parents can tolerate the shame triggered by the adolescent's various humiliating behaviours; they do not react as quickly and as harshly to shaming messages from the teen.
- The parents experience more empathy towards their child. Parents feel that they 'see' their child in a different way.

The adolescent is not therefore the sole beneficiary of this intervention. Parents also change, learning that they can emancipate themselves from their patterned shame reactions to the child's shameless behaviours.

The second type of intervention to counter shamelessness is the 'public opinion' intervention (Omer, *et al*, 2004). The rational for using this intervention rests on the assumption that, just as the others' presence can create shame, it also has the power to ameliorate it.

The public (that is any outsider who is aware of the individual's behaviours) plays a major role in the development and maintenance of the experience of shame, as shame is an emotion that has to do with how we are perceived by others (Gilbert, 2007) and with the experience of being exposed. This is the reason why, in situations of crisis and escalating conflict, family members tend to involve fewer people and become more private and isolated. In such situations, the public and its opinions are not perceived as a resource but rather as a source of criticism and blame, which can increase the shame for family members. This is exactly the process that is challenged and reversed in NVR.

In the public opinion intervention we use the power of the public to regulate shame through two combined actions: (a) 'going public': when information which is shame related is shared with other people outside the family, and (b) bringing the public: when people outside the family get in touch with the adolescent and reveal that they know about the events within the family.

Both of these actions expose the adolescent to shame and therefore must be planned carefully. This leads to a different kind of experience – a controllable exposure to the emotion of shame, which maximises the potential of the public for shame management while reducing potential negative shaming processes.

The ability to speak out and voice private matters is an essential part of the process of empowerment and shame regulation (Sanderson, 2015). In going public, parents are coached in sharing the shameful behaviours of their child with other people who are, crucially, supportive. After sharing their experiences with others, parents request these supporters to contact the child and deliver a message to him or her. This parental strategy of openness and transparency is announced to the child ahead of time in a respectful way.

The messages that these supportive friends and family members should deliver to the child (via phone, email and letters) are short, concise and are composed of three parts: revealing knowledge, expressing an opinion and de-shaming. For example, a message delivered to John, an adolescent boy, after an incident in which he pushed his mother might take the following form:

Revealing knowledge – 'I heard that you pushed your mother last night.'

Expressing an opinion – 'That's not the John I know' or, 'That's not right'.

De-shaming – 'What happened?' or, 'I care about you and your family and I still think you are a good person. Let me know if I can help'.

Such messages have been found to be very effective in reducing aggressive and disrespectful behaviours (Weinblatt & Omer, 2008). For children who are disconnected from shame, the involvement of social networks in this way arouses shame and brings it to the level where it can perform its original, healthy function – inhibiting hurtful behaviours towards others. What follows after such messages are actions of moving closer and reconnecting with the child (checking up on him or her, eating something together, playing computer games). This resembles what Braithwaite (1989) calls 're-integrative shaming', a process of justice making in which shaming is followed by efforts to reintegrate the offender back into the community. This is exactly the opposite process of stigmatisation, which implies a disintegrative shaming process in which the offender (in our case, an adolescent) is rejected by others.

For many families, such public involvement is not an easy task. Parents and children who are involved in intense conflicts often have a great deal to hide. Parents can feel ashamed of their parenting, ashamed of their child's behaviour, ashamed of needing help, and ashamed of their helplessness. The child often feels ashamed of his failures, commonly social and academic in nature, ashamed of receiving negative attention, ashamed of his weak parents and ashamed of his own behaviours.

The decision in families as to what may become public and what should remain private is thus constantly negotiated. It is usually shame that constructs and signifies the boundary between what is private and what is public. As shame grows, private life becomes more dominant, keeping the relationships with other people at a distance. As this dynamic intensifies, the attitudes of others become threatening and dangerous, leading to more alienation, isolation and shame, which in turn puts more obstacles in the way of people using their support systems in helpful ways.

In NVR we challenge this process through interventions that renegotiate the boundary between the private and the public and ultimately lead to improvements in the regulation of shame.

In the process of introducing supportive others into family life and adopting a policy of openness, the parents and child need to overcome the fear of being shamed by others from their social network (Weinblatt, 2013). These fears include:

- **The shame of needing help.** For many people in many different cultures, needing help is perceived as shameful. Needing help and not receiving it is even worse. Parents often fear that their appeals for help from others will be denied. Overcoming this obstacle is crucial for the shame regulation process.
- **The shame of failing.** There is no assurance that involving others will change the dynamic between parent and child. Parents who are already experiencing a sense of defeat do not need another disappointment in their lives, a let-down that will only shame them more.
- **The tyranny of the majority.** Public opinion can be an instrument for inducing social control and enforcing conformity. Indeed, anthropologists have

 

identified 'shame cultures' that use shame as the main tool for maintaining order (Benedict, 1954). In these cultures, people fear public humiliation and shame, and their behaviour is governed by the need to avoid it.

- **The shame of stigma.** Parents feel that 'going public' will potentially stigmatise the child and will lead others to reject them. They are also concerned that they will be stigmatised themselves as 'bad' parents, incompetent and weak.

These are serious issues that need to be handled carefully. Exposing what is going on at home should always be done in a collaborative spirit with the parents. Such a sensitive approach allows the teen as well the parents to get in touch with their shame in a way that is not destructive but that leads to a greater acceptance of themselves, their weaknesses and their vulnerabilities.

# Conclusion

In intense family conflicts it is common for adolescents to shift from being in states of shamefulness to states of shamelessness. In NVR, the combined interventions to regulate both unregulated shame states leads to more emotional stability for all family members. For mitigating feelings of shame, the therapist helps family members replace negative and harmful shame by using respectful and compassionate interactions that promote better shame regulation and a healthier relationship with shame. For shamelessness, the therapist promotes experiences of controlled exposure to reintegrate shame when absent.

## References


Benedict R (1946) *The Chrysanthemum and the Sword. Patterns of Japanese Culture*. Boston: Houghton Mifflin.

Braithwaite J (1989) *Crime, Shame and Reintegration*. Cambridge University Press.

DeYoung PA (2015) *Understanding and Treating Chronic Shame: A relational / neurobiological approach*. Abingdon: Routledge.

Gilbert P (2007) The evolution of shame as a marker for relationship security: A biopsychosocial approach. In: JL Tracy, RW Robins & JP Tangney (Eds) *The Self-Conscious Emotions: Theory and research* (pp283–309). New York: Guilford Press.

Gilligan J (2001) *Violence: A reflection on the national epidemic*. New York: Pantheon.

Greenberg LS & Goldman RN (2008) *Emotion-focused Couples Therapy: The dynamics of emotion, love, and power*. American Psychological Association.

Kaufman G (1996) *The Psychology of Shame: Theory and treatment of shame-based syndrome (2nd ed)*. New York: Springer.

Nathanson DL (1992) *Shame and Pride: Affect, sex, and the birth of the self*. WW Norton & Company.

Omer H (2001) Helping Parents Deal with Children's Acute Disciplinary Problems Without Escalation: The Principle of Nonviolent Resistance. *Family Process* **40** (1) 53–66.

Omer H, Weinblatt U & Kerwinkel C (2004) The parent manual. In: H Omer *Non-Violent Resistance: A new approach to violent and self-destructive children*. Cambridge University Press.

Sanderson C (2015) *Counselling Skills for Working with Shame*. Jessica Kingsley Publishers.

Scheff TJ (1997) *Emotions, the social bond, and human reality: Part/whole analysis*. Cambridge University Press.

Tangney JP & Dearing RL (2002) *Shame and Guilt*. New York, NY: Guilford Press.

Tangney JP, Stuewig J & Mashek D (2007) Moral emotions and moral behavior. *Annual Review of Psychology* **58** 345–372.

Tomkins S (1963) *Affect/imagery/consciousness. Vol. 2: The negative affects*. Oxford: England Springer.

Weinblatt U & Omer H (2008) Nonviolent resistance: a treatment for parents of children with acute behavior problems. *Journal of Marital and Family Therapy* **34** (1) 75–92.

Weinblatt U (2013) Die Regulierung des Schamgefühls bei intensiven Eltern-Kind-Konflikten: Praktiken des gewaltlosen Widerstands, die die Öffentlichkeit einbeziehen (Regulating shame in intense parent – child conflict through public opinion interventions in NVR therapy). *Familiendynamik: Systemische Praxis und Forschung* **38** (1) 62–71.

Weinblatt U (2016) *Die Nähe ist ganz nah! Scham und Verletzungen in Beziehungen überwinden*. Vandenhoeck & Ruprecht.

 

# Chapter 2: Improving fathers' engagement and collaboration between parents

**By Naama Gershy, PhD and Haim Omer, PhD**

## Introduction

Numerous studies over the past 30 years have emphasised the contribution of fathers to child development and the importance of engaging fathers in raising their children. Despite these studies, many clinicians struggle to get fathers to engage effectively with their children's upbringing and many are still absent from parenting interventions. This chapter describes strategies for engaging fathers and for improving collaboration between parents.

## Context

A major challenge encountered by counsellors working with parents is improving the level of collaboration between them. Several things can exacerbate the problem such as one of the parents (often the father) showing no interest in treatment, high levels of parental dispute, contradictory parenting ideologies about education and/or discipline, or parents blaming one another for the child's problems. In the past, these challenges have led many counsellors to argue that couple therapy is required before any improvement in parenting can take place.

We think this is problematic for a number of reasons:

1. Couple therapy is a complex and often unpredictable process. Making couple therapy a condition for parenting guidance can prevent them from taking action to improve their parenting. The child is meanwhile left to continue in their problematic situation until the couple's problems are solved.

2. Management of their child's behaviours is often a major cause of parental disputes. In such cases, parenting interventions can help both the child and the parents, even if other sources of conflict between the couple are not directly addressed.
3. Most parents are motivated to improve the child's condition regardless of the difficulties in their relationship with one another. This motivation is often stronger than the willingness to improve their relationship.

Although general couple therapy is therefore not useful, specifically improving co-operation between parents in relation to their child can be, and in our experience even a modest improvement in parental co-operation can bring about meaningful consequences for the parenting system. For example, parents can learn to stop undermining each other even if they disagree, which can help a child experience the world as less chaotic. Furthermore, even a modest reduction in arguments and blame between parents, can help them pay more attention to their parenting practices and to feel more confident executing new practices they have learned in therapy. When parents realise that minor steps can bring improvements, they are usually more willing to take the next steps.

# Theory and literature

## Fathers' involvement

It is usually mothers who initiate first contact with counselling services and who schedule the first treatment appointment. In families in which the father is less involved in childcare or works long hours, some mothers ask if meetings can take place without him. Furthermore, mothers are still perceived by many counsellors as the primary caregiver in childcare, and the one treatment should focus on.

Given these facts, it is no wonder that many fathers consider therapy to be less relevant than mothers do, or that they are often reluctant to join therapy. While some fathers express their reluctance directly when invited to participate, more often they express it by missing appointments, taking a passive role and not following treatment recommendations.

This absence of fathers from their child's treatment is concerning given the growing evidence in the developmental literature for the importance of a father's role in their child's development, as well as in treatment success (Lamb & Lewis, 2010; Phares *et al*, 2010). A father's refusal to participate in treatment, or their early drop out, were found to be related to reduced improvement in child behaviour following treatment (Carr, 1998) and to difficulty in maintaining treatment gains (Bagner & Eyberg, 2003; Webster-Stratton *et al*, 2004).

 

A father's contribution to parenting mainly occurs through two main paths: his own direct role in taking care of the child himself, and his ability to support the mother's parenting. For children with behaviour problems, it is this ability to support the mother that is of particular importance. In such families, mothers are often the ones who bear the bulk of the negative interactions and conflicts with the child (Lavi-Levavi *et al*, 2013). Studies indicate that the capacity of mothers to cope with their child's special needs or aggression grows when she receives support from her immediate support network, and in particular the support of the father. Mothers that feel isolated and unappreciated often struggle more to exert their authority over their child (DeKlyen *et al*, 1998; Suárez & Baker, 1997).

# Description of NVR therapy practice

To understand and enhance fathers' involvement and collaboration in therapy, we conducted an analysis of NVR therapy cases in which fathers had been successfully and unsuccessfully involved (Gershy & Omer, 2017). The study drew a number of practical conclusions.

## Insisting on including fathers from the beginning

In NVR, the father's presence and participation in treatment is of the highest priority. We emphasise this from the first telephone contact. If the mother makes contact and says that the father is not interested or is too busy to come, we insist that he comes at least to the first meeting. If the mother expresses difficulty in convincing the father, we ask for her reasons. If the main reason is the father's lack of interest or involvement, we ask to discuss this directly with him on the phone and we explain that involving the father is essential, even if only to inform him about the treatment process and goals.

This clarification almost always leads the mother to agree that we can contact the father. This is a crucial moment, as even a passive consent from our side that counselling can take place without the father means we are collaborating with a situation that has the potential to harm the child.

## Emphasising the importance of the fathers' point of view and promoting an action-based discourse

There are several points that should be emphasised to the father in order to enhance his participation:

- That he is a full participant in the child's education and that his point of view is essential for our understanding of the child's difficulties.

- That fathers see things differently to mothers, partly because they have more perspective and are frequently less absorbed in the daily hassles of child care.
- That our goal is to strengthen both parents, to reduce their isolation, and to help them feel more protected, supported and more effective.
- The father must come to the first meeting at least. If the father continues to express disinterest we emphasise that we respect his decision but we ask for his permission to inform him about the steps we will take in relation to the child. If he is willing, once in a while, we will ask him to express support for those actions he agrees with.

Many fathers respond positively to our practical approach and to our emphasis on parental strength. Most fathers are interested in receiving treatment updates and respond positively to our requests. Such positive responses signal that the father's attitude towards treatment has improved, at least by some small degree, e.g. from rejection to a neutral/curious attitude, or from neutrality to an attitude of modest support. Such modest improvements may be a sign of other positive changes to come.

## Case study: Yoav

Yoav, a 14-year-old boy, used to curse and physically attack his mother every time she did not comply with his demands. The father was aware of his wife's difficulties with Yoav but was absent from the house most of the day and did not experience the violence directly.

Upon hearing about the treatment plan the father placed a veto on the recruitment of supporters. 'In our culture,' he said, 'we solve our own problems. The dirty laundry stays in the home.' The counsellor did not argue with the father, focusing instead on the mother's experiences of abuse from her son, who described her fear and desperation which led her at times to entertain thoughts of suicide.

Yoav's mother felt supported by her husband's sense of outrage at the boy's behaviour and by the fact that the counsellor and the father agreed that that the situation was very serious and needed to change. Due to the extent of the violence, the counsellor was able to say, 'This is a very serious problem and your wife will need all available help to stop the violence. In our experience, problems of this magnitude require a large and strong task force. Who would you like to recruit so we could give your wife the support she deserves?' The father initially agreed to recruit one supporter, but gradually invited additional ones.

The practical, concrete and non-blaming language of the counsellor enabled the father to change his position and eventually to agree to treatment acts which he had initially opposed.

 

## Gradually involving the father in tasks related to the child

A father's disinterest in joining therapy is sometimes related to his generally low involvement in childcare. He may be unaware of the difficulties, feel marginalised in the decision making process, or feel that his advice is rarely listened to and it is therefore useless to get involved. Such fathers may respond positively to more gradual attempts to involve them, provided that the attempts are not too demanding or the father is not expected to share the load equally with the mother (these goals can be too threatening for fathers who are used to playing a minimal role in family life).

We believe in looking for small opportunities for positive contact between them and the child. Sometimes the parents can agree on a focused task that the father can undertake and can help lift some of the burden from the mother's shoulders. For example, they might take responsibility for putting the child to bed, or driving the children to school in the morning. A well-defined task can help the father experience a sense of success. However, finding the right task is not easy and requires assessing what tasks the fathers can contribute to without being expected to dive in at the deep end. In addition, one needs to make sure that the mother is willing to accept a limited effort by the father. Sometimes the mother is so angry at the father that she prefers to forego his services all together. The counsellor has to co-ordinate the father's involvement diplomatically and in a way that feels safe for both parents.

It is important to emphasise that the father's first steps are intended to be limited. Again, if we try to push a father to become fully involved too early, we risk losing the little he is willing to give. The counsellor should therefore be attentive to the mother's disappointment that the bulk of the burden will remain hers, or to her frustration that the father receives positive regard from the counsellor for doing so little. The mother's disappointment can become an obstacle preventing her from appreciating the changes the father is making. A disparaging remark by the mother can sometime push the father away and the counsellor should pay attention and address this possibility by acknowledging both the mother's frustration and the father's emerging willingness.

## Working with authoritarian fathers

The difficulty in engaging a father is sometimes due to his authoritarian attitude which can cause the mother to worry about his harsh or aggressive reactions towards the child. In the eyes of these fathers, reacting with patience means that the child has 'won'. However, our experience has taught us that authoritative and coercive parenting cannot be addressed through discussions about love and acceptance. Though it may seem paradoxical, in these cases the counsellor's emphasis on parental *strength* is crucial and may help decrease the father's resistance. For example, 'We strive for real strength; a strength that will manifest in your ability to stop submitting to your child's demands, to feel active, competent and legitimated in front of his aggressive behaviours. Both you and your child will realise that you are much stronger than you used to be.'

Many counsellors worry that expressing such a position to an authoritarian or impulsive father may support his problematic approach to discipline. However, a major component of these discussions about strength concerns issues of self-control. We explain to impulsive fathers that their outbursts of temper actually lower the level of respect they receive from their children. For those fathers who tend to react with physical aggression, we add something along the following lines:

> *'I'm afraid that you're in great danger. If, for example, the school counsellor notices that your child has been physically hurt, your angry outbursts and aggression may come to light and you may find yourself in trouble with the law. We need to prevent this from happening and we will teach you to be strong in a positive way without putting yourself in danger.'*

Speaking directly to fathers about the consequences of their behaviours while highlighting parental strength may allow engagement with even a very authoritarian or violent father.

## Working with overprotective or spoiling fathers

Generally speaking, and certainly in the past, fathers have often taken a more authoritarian role than mothers, serving as the source of discipline for a child. Today that situation is sometimes reversed. Divorced fathers, for instance, often view their relationships with their children as fragile, and they therefore strive to maintain a harmonious and pleasant relationship by avoiding any confrontations. If the father is concerned about losing his child's affection, he may resist collaborating with 'unpopular' steps (for example, the sit in, telephone round or the recruitment of supporters). In the sample in our study, this tendency was less common for divorced mothers.

This is another situation in which the counsellor should proceed with small steps that do not require the father to change his position too dramatically or too quickly. For example, the father might be convinced to tell the child he is no longer willing to reverse the mother's decisions but will uphold them instead, or to explain that he will no longer make agreements with the child behind the mother's back.

 

In itself, such a step will not significantly change the father's spoiling or overprotective behaviour, but it may improve the parents' collaboration with one another, replacing the previous coalition between father and child that undermined the mother's position.

At times, a father may be willing to take bigger steps, for example when he agrees to take part in a sit-in together with the mother. The counsellor can help to encourage this by making it clear that the father's contribution can be meaningful even if he does not see things eye to eye with the mother. Actually, the father's support is even more significant if he does not identify with the mother's position because it shows the child that their previous coalition with their father is over.

## Acknowledging the mothers' hard work

Mothers who carry the burden of childcare need recognition for their hard work. A father's lack of acknowledgement of the mother's role can make it difficult for the mother to appreciate what may initially be small changes the father is willing to make. In our study, we often witnessed mothers giving their partners the cold shoulder, or resenting the father's attempts to become more involved. Some of the mothers felt anger towards the counsellor for praising the father's minor efforts. Some counsellors interpreted this reaction of the mother as a reflection of her own emotional needs and her desire to maintain her control over what happens at home and over the relationship with the child.

In our experience, however, reluctance on the mother's part can be much diminished if the counsellor openly expresses recognition and praise for her hard work. For example, the counsellor can reframe the mother's disappointment as a consequence of the deep inequality in the burden of father and mother. Such a statement may reduce the mother's reluctance and help the father to accept her protests.

### Case study

Alma, a 10-year-old girl, suffered from a rare skin disease that required intensive treatment and a high level of parental monitoring. Almas's father worked long hours and her mother was solely responsible for Alma's care. Nevertheless, her parents arrived together at treatment following Alma's refusal to take her medications which caused much friction between her and her mother. The counsellor assumed that Alma's opposition was related to a power struggle between her and her mother. He therefore suggested that the father should take some of the responsibility over Alma's medical care and 'free' the mother from being the only one in charge. The father agreed.

In the following therapy meeting, Alma's father reported that the plan had worked nicely. Alma had collaborated with his care and had been less oppositional during the week. The therapist expressed his appreciation for Alma's father's willingness to take up this role, and expressed his satisfaction at the quick change in Alma's behaviour. Alma's mother, however, was less enthusiastic, criticising her husband for taking shortcuts and not following the medical directions closely enough.

Alma's father was hurt by this criticism and felt ready to give up. To resolve the situation, the therapist said:

> *'I understand that something new happened in the family this week. Like every new thing, it will take time and repetition to turn it from a one time event into a habit. You, [mother], have been taking care of Alma by yourself for many years, dealing everyday with the difficulties involved in her severe medical condition and with her resistance. You've sacrificed a lot to take care of her. You carried the burden for many years, until you felt this is not a job for one person. You, [father], made the first step towards becoming more involved in Alma's treatment. This important step showed that you are serious and ready to join [mother's] team. However, this is only a first step. For this step to become meaningful we need you, [mother], to remember that what you have learned through many years of hard work cannot be learned in one week. Will you be willing to teach [father] gradually how to help you take care of Alma? Will you [father] be willing that [mother] teaches you what she has learned?'*

## When should the mother be seen alone?

The steps we have described to engage the father can reduce the imbalance in parental involvement, maximising the benefits that each parent can provide. However, there will be times when the father's attitude will remain negative and critical despite all efforts to engage him positively. In one of the cases in our sample, after repeated attempts to re-engage the father, we reached the conclusion that the attempts had misfired and it was highly unlikely that he would ever co-operate. We realised that continuing to invest our efforts in the father's engagement was leaving the mother alone, not only at home but also in treatment. After consulting with the mother, we decided to tell the father:

> *'On several occasions you have told us that the only one who needs help is your wife, since she is the one who is dissatisfied and suffers most from clashes with your daughter. There's no doubt that she needs help more than you do, given the higher responsibility she carries at home. We therefore*

 

*agree with you and will continue working with your wife alone. You don't have to come to the meetings, but we will be glad to update you by mail. Your views remain important to us, so we'll be happy to hear your thoughts in future and tell you what we are working on.'*

This message worked well. The mother felt justified and supported, and the treatment progressed much better with her than when the father had been present. Surprisingly, the father's readiness to co-operate actually increased when the treatment was defined as 'helping his wife deal with her difficulties'. He responded well to the mail updates and collaborated with the treatment steps better than during the joint counselling.

## Summary

One of the main conditions for a successful intervention is an accurate evaluation of the father's involvement in the child's life, and an assessment of the level of support between the parents. Such an evaluation helps the counsellor adapt the therapeutic tasks to the father's level of involvement and to help the couple increase their collaboration, taking into account their baseline level of co-operation and support.

The literature on paternal drop-out from parent counselling (Fabiano, 2007; Lundahl, Tollefson *et al*, 2008; Panter-Brick *et al*, 2014) shows that it does not take much to make fathers feel unwelcome or marginalised. The counsellor should remember that the goal of their intervention is not to turn an absent and uninvolved father into a full partner, nor is it to transform highly conflicted parents into a smoothly functioning team. The goal is first and foremost to help the parents, and the father in particular, to have a positive experience of growing collaboration and involvement.

Our experience at the NVR clinic at Schneider Hospital in Israel has taught us that training counsellors to think about the engagement of fathers as an important therapeutic task, and teaching the basic engagement principles described above, can dramatically increase the rates at which fathers engage during therapy.

## References

Bagner DM & Eyberg SM (2003). Father involvement in parent training: when does it matter? *Journal of Clinical Child & Adolescent Psychology* **32** (4) 599–605 doi: 10.1207/S15374424JCCP3204_13.

Carr A (1998) The inclusion of fathers in family therapy: a research based perspective. *Contemporary Family Therapy* **20** (3) 371–383 doi: 10.1023/A:1022425231125.

DeKlyen M, Speltz M & Greenberg M (1998) Fathering and early onset conduct problems: positive and negative parenting, father–son attachment, and the marital context. *Clinical Child and Family*

*Psychology Review* **1** (1) 3–21 doi: 10.1023/A:1021844214633.

Fabiano GA (2007) Father participation in behavioral parent training for ADHD: Review and recommendations for increasing inclusion and engagement. *Journal of Family Psychology* **21** (4) 683–693.

Gershy N & Omer H (2017) Engaging fathers in parent training: a qualitative study. *Journal of Family Psychotherapy* **28** (1) 38–58 doi: 10.1080/08975353.2017.1283143.

Lamb ME & Lewis C (2010) The development and significance of father–child relationships in two-parent families. In: ME Lamb (Ed) *The Role of the Father in Child Development* (pp94–153). Hoboken, NJ, US: John Wiley & Sons Inc.

Lavi-Levavi I, Shachar I & Omer H (2013) Training in nonviolent resistance for parents of violent children: differences between fathers and mothers. *Journal of Systemic Therapies* **32** (4) 79–93 doi: 10.1521/jsyt.2013.32.4.79.

Lundahl BW, Tollefson D, Risser H & Lovejoy MC (2008) A meta-analysis of father involvement in parent training. *Research on Social Work Practice* **18** (2) 97–106. doi: 10.1177/1049731507309828.

Panter-Brick C, Burgess A, Eggerman M, McAllister F, Pruett K & Leckman JF (2014). Practitioner review: engaging fathers – recommendations for a game change in parenting interventions based on a systematic review of the global evidence. *Journal of Child Psychology and Psychiatry* **55** (11) 1187–1212 doi: 10.1111/jcpp.12280.

Patterson GR & Maccoby EE (1980) Mothers: the unacknowledged victims. *Monographs of the Society for Research in Child Development* **45** (5) 1–64. doi: 10.2307/1165841.

Phares V, Rojas A, Thurston IB & Hankinson JC (2010) Including fathers in clinical interventions for children and adolescents. In: ME Lamb (Ed) *The Role of the Father in child development.* Hoboken, NJ, US: John Wiley & Sons Inc..

Suárez LM & Baker BL (1997) Child externalizing behavior and parents' stress: the role of social support. *Family Relations* **46** (4) 373–381 doi: 10.2307/585097.

Webster-Stratton C, Reid MJ & Hammond M (2004) Treating children with early-onset conduct problems: Intervention outcomes for parent, child, and teacher training. *Journal of Clinical Child and Adolescent Psychology* **33** (1) 105–124 doi: 10.1207/S15374424JCCP3301_11.

 

# Chapter 3: Fathering and NVR: changing relationships, engagement and perceptions

**By Julia Jude and Veronica Rivera-Gould**

> *'All individuals, regardless of gender, must be encouraged to see themselves as both caregivers and financial providers – and be supported in both these roles.'* (Heilman *et al*, 2017, p1)

## Introduction

The significance of the debate concerning fathers' involvement in parent training suggests that fathers play an important role that should not be overlooked, but rather they should be encouraged to participate. Given the overwhelming weight of evidence that we now have from research and literature confirming the value of fathers' participation, this is recognised in the non-violent resistance (NVR) parent-training approach, whereby the attendance of the whole family, including the fathers, is meaningful.

However, this is not a practice that is taken up in many parenting training programmes locally, nationally or internationally (Heilman *et al*, 2017). As a result, practitioners and clinicians are being invited to find numerous ways and methods of working with and engaging fathers. As authors working in children services, we were aware that fathers were scarcely mentioned in case notes, referral discussions or in reviews. As a result they became 'invisible', a situation that clinicians accepted without challenge. The consequences of accepting this dominant narrative – that fathers are not entitled to be asked, encouraged or informed about what was going on with their child/children – created a context in which clinicians unintentionally ignored aspects of a father's responsibility, duty and role, making them effectively redundant in parenting their children.

This chapter explores the literature on fathering and argues that professionals should be taking greater steps to make fathers more visible in the day-to-day aspects of their children's development and well-being. We reflect on the results from a pilot study conducted by the authors that explored what it means for fathers to be involved in their children's lives through their attendance and participation in a multi-parent NVR group. We argue that professionals and services need to be more invested in supporting fathers in their parental role and identity in order to enable both mothers and fathers to become invested in a co-parental relationship for the betterment of their children's lives. Furthermore, we argue that further research is needed to understand the nature of the support fathers need to fulfil this role, and how parenting training might better meet their needs.

## The impact of fatherhood and attachment theories

Several researchers (Flouri & Buchanan, 2003; Horn & Sylvester, 2002; Pfiffner *et al*, 2001; Allen & Daly, 2007) note that children of involved fathers tend to have more positive social relationships with their peers, and their relational responses tend to be characterised by less aggression and conflict, with more co-operative, more caring, and more considered relational qualities. Furthermore, a father's level of involvement has been shown to directly impact on adolescent experiences and well-being and there is a positive connection between fathers' involvement and many aspects of child and adolescent development. Heilman *et al*'s (2017) analysis of 700 studies across the world notes that effective parent training that includes fathers can achieve multiple objectives, including a reduction in many forms of violence and an increase in the father's involvement in childcare. Furthermore, they argue that although including fathers in treatment plans in family work is demonstrably effective, the availability of these treatments is scarce.

Theories on child development (Bee & Boyd, 2014; Bronfenbrenner, 1979) suggest that positive experiences of fathering are supported by positive experiences of having been fathered effectively during one's own childhood. Yet attachment theories (Van IJzendoorn *et al*, 1995; Fernald, 1985) appear to erase the presence of fathers in the early experiences of their children's lives, tending instead to focus solely on the roles of mothers (Lamb, 2004). For example, Bowlby's (1997) and Ainsworth *et al*'s (1978) work on attachment illuminated the connections between maternal loss and deprivation and the development of personality disorders and poor emotional security. Their theory of attachment is deemed to provide a universal framework for child development and is one of the most applied conceptual structures for understanding how individuals self-regulate their emotions. Their work argues that a child's development of feelings of control and their sense of security stems from the infant-mother relationship and appears to be significant in the regulation of affect, the establishment of other social relationships and the child's ability to negotiate and co-ordinate tasks. Furthermore, this theory posits that the child's principal relationship with their mother will influence and affect all other relationships they create and engage in. Importantly, this influence continues throughout the child's developmental cycle and into adulthood.

But not everyone is in agreement with the ideas of attachment theory. Krause and Maitra (2014) argue that the attachment model is too Eurocentric, as it supports a predominantly Western European structure of parenting, which is assumed to represent a universal model, while failing to acknowledge that the contextual, cultural patterns and experiences of child rearing are not universal. In addition, Harris *et al* (1998) dismisses the view that parents have a significant impact over their child's personality, arguing instead that the child's friendship group and peers have greater influences on them than their parents. Field *et al* (1995), meanwhile, suggests that the child can have significant figures other than the mother. But more importantly, children show their attachment to different people in different ways, influenced by the nature of their relationship with that person. This is relevant to communities where the extended family have a greater role in child rearing. For example, Richter and Morrel's work (2006) demonstrates that indigenous fathers in South Africa were as invested in child rearing as mothers and yet they are often overlooked in all aspects of scholarly work and literature on child development and child rearing.

So, how do fathers act as positive role models and offer positive experiences of fathering when their roles and experiences have been excluded from theories and knowledge and that inform our thinking as professionals?

Green (2012) argues that it is not by accident that the main care figures are mothers, not fathers. Many feminist scholars have argued that motherhood and mothering are not natural pathways for women but that they are historically, culturally and socially constructed, claiming that the dominant discourse ascribes the parenting role to women rather than men. O'Reilly (2008) concurs with this view, arguing that policy shapes the way women manage their lives through the way provisions are delivered, which may create opportunities for women or restrict their choices. Green (2012) maintains that it suits society to make women more visible and responsible in the parenting role, while making men less visible and responsible, since they are deemed to be needed at work and that mothers need to be present in the early stages of childhood.

Lawler (2000) suggests that this construction is driven by a capitalist drive to increase productivity and economic growth rather than meeting the needs of mothers or fathers and their children. Lamb (2004) does not disagree with this perspective, but argues that our attention needs to be focused on workplace practices and organisational cultures, which impact on child rearing, alleging that policies and procedures in the workplace are often barriers to fathers' involvement in family life. Lamb (2004) suggests that public and private sector employers have not made it easy for fathers to become involved in their children's care and that they respond in way that excludes them.

Lee and Duxbury (1998) argue that workplaces should move towards providing more support for fathers, including paternity leave and more flexible working arrangements. However, Milkie and Peltola's (1999) research highlighted that fathers were often less likely to take advantage of flexible working and parenting leave. Once again, it could be argued that more needs to be done to enable fathers to feel that they are entitled to access support services when they are provided, and more research is needed to explore the workplace barriers preventing fathers' involvement in family life.

## Big boys don't cry: sacred cows, myths and truths of male views and experiences of therapy

Addis and Mahalik (2003) suggest that fathers' invisibility at home and their absence in child rearing has created a context in which men are also absent when their child requires psychological support from outside agencies. They claim that there is still a notion of masculinity that seems to suggest that men and psychological interventions don't go together. According to Addis and Mahalik (2003), fathers are only dragged to therapy when there is a crisis in their lives. They argue that this is associated with a negative attitude towards psychological support stemming from early childhood and the ways in which boys are conditioned. Good *et al* (2005) argue that men have become confused about their role in society and have little control over their lives and the lives of their children, and thus have become destructive both to themselves and others. They argue that what it means to be masculine has changed and continues to change – socially, economically, and in terms of race and ethnicity. This has resulted in men not knowing how to 'be' or what to be. In order for men to enter therapy, the field needs to demonstrate that it understands their issues.

Jordan *et al* (2012) conclude that agencies working with men need to do more to include them and to accommodate their emotional needs. Services need to be more proactive around access and outreach, and may be more engaging if they are not exclusively related to mental health but also to social community-service groups. They refer to the stigma attached to men who seek help and the expectations for males to be strong and not need support. Consistent attendance is, they say, a sign of having a good experience with services, and hearing the testimonies of others improved attendance and outcomes. Jordan *et al* (2012) state that clinicians' attitudes are crucial in building rapport and engaging fathers in treatment.

The situation seems to be somewhat different in America, where research suggests that many black men are more willing to enter therapy. Thorn and Sarata (1998) also found that black men and women from lower socio-economic groups often seek therapeutic support. They argue that racism and self-esteem are two of the main reasons for this, while Boyd-Franklin and Franklin (2000) say, '*Raising African American sons is one of the greatest challenges on the face of the earth. Worry goes with the landscape but if we are to make a difference for our young men we must follow the words of the Ashanti proverb... "you must act as if it is impossible to fail".*'

The authors describe the importance of love in bringing up black boys, and argue that the value of fathers cannot be overestimated. This perspective on fathering is especially pertinent to black men, according to Ball (2009), who are the most socially excluded of any community which, she argues, is as a result of colonial interventions that have disrupted indigenous families and communities.

## Making fathering our business

As authors, our anecdotal experience of working with fathers across cultures is limited when compared to our experience of working with mothers. The absence of fathers in treatment with their families was not an area that we questioned in our clinical practice. Instead, we came to accept this invisibility as part of our usual practice.

Change occurred through our practice (Jude & Rivera-Gould, 2014) facilitating a multi-parent group (Day & Heismann, 2010), which provided a conjoined service for child and adolescent mental health service (CAMHS) users and users of children's services. The group ran for ten weeks, during which parents explored the main presenting difficulty or behaviour of their child, and each week they reviewed NVR principles as a way of understanding their child's behaviour and the application of the idea to their parenting style. In addition, parents were invited to reflect and engage in discussions that aimed to repair their relationships.

In the three consecutive years of facilitating such groups, we noticed that certain fathers would attend every session and complete the group, which was unusual in our experience. This surprised and delighted us, and created a desire in us to understand their motives.

We therefore decided to undertake a pilot study with seven fathers who had attended the groups (by 'fathers', we refer to men who have taken on the responsibility of participating in bringing up a young person). During the interviews for this study, the fathers received information about the importance of participation, follow up, and completion. What follows are some of the highlights and responses from two participants (one of white British and the other of Asian descent).

### How did you become involved in the group?

'It was my social worker who involved us in the group. We wish we were offered it before but it wasn't offered. When she called us in we thought, yeah... we'll go.'

'I would give anything a try.'

### What made you come to the group?

'To get a better relationship with my daughter.'

'I was having problems with my son... and I found that no matter how hard I tried, communication wasn't being made.'

### What was your initial feeling when presented with the idea of non-violent resistance?

'When it was first presented to me, I didn't want to come; this was not for me.'

'When I first heard of it, I wasn't too keen.'

### What was your initial feeling when arriving at the first group session?

'I didn't want to talk at all. I don't even talk to people at work... but when I got there, yeah, I found it easier.'

### Do you remember what you were thinking?

'I didn't think of anything bad, I didn't think there was much to talk about, 'cause it's gone on for years... we just have to get on with it... but I did get something from it.'

'Initially when you came to my house, it was mostly women, so immediately we [men] are taking a step back, and you say hold on a minute this is a woman thing, let her deal with it, that was my house issue. However, I'll always look for proof, so if someone says this system works then I would say, "look, I can't say it does or it doesn't unless I've tried it".'

'Meeting people who have similar problems, and when they talk about it and you start to talk about it, it makes things easier. You can say something without feeling embarrassed or someone judging me.'

### Can you tell me how it was to speak in front of other people who were not your own family about your problem?

'It was a massive step… yeah, it was a massive step. It felt as if everyone's story was the same and that we were all in the same situation. I couldn't speak with someone if you have never experienced it… It wouldn't be worth speaking to someone because they wouldn't know where I am coming from.'

### What made you complete the programme?

'It worked, I saw results.'

'It's what's at the end of the tunnel. Isn't it? Why would anybody want to complete anything if you don't see what the results are. You start something; you must see the result at the end of it. Why do something halfway and then say it didn't work? I was enjoying it; it was all right. It was fun.'

These statements established that the fathers were interested in and concerned by the difficulties experienced by their children, and invested in resolving them. They overcame their initial doubts about the programme and their fears and uncertainties of being in a group setting; they engaged in the group work, they trusted other parents and the group facilitators while sharing their personal stories. They also accepted the support and guidance offered by the group, which included changes in some of their parenting approaches. The statements regarding their completion of the group expose their willingness to complete something they had started, and, above all, how their motivation to complete the group was increased after seeing positive results – their children were responding to their parenting strategies.

In some of the literature reviewed, there was an assumption that men were simply not interested in therapy or in talking to resolve the relationship issues in their families, but the fathers we interviewed had an alternative explanation. They suggested that the idea that men shied away from talking showed a degree of naivety and claimed that the issue was more than 'just talking'. They explained that some of their ambivalence about accessing services was connected to the fear and shame of having to talk so openly about the troubles they were having with their children, and their sense of failure, of wounded pride. This connects to ideas expressed by Cowan and Cowan (2003) and O'Reilly's (2008) ideas regarding the role of dominant discourses in shaping our construction of fathering and masculinity. They argue that change requires contexts in which ideas and dialogue can be transformed into practice. Fathers told us that what kept them coming to the group were the tools they acquired which they could use with their children, test out, reflect upon, and then give feedback on their experiences to the group.

Borrowing from Lamb (2004), we argue that fathers' ambivalence about entering therapy might be more about how they are invited to talk. Perhaps we need to know more about what we don't know. What we do know is that the fathers we spoke to have feelings, which are not signs of weakness but are signs of simply being human, and this approach seems to encourage men to talk about them.

Fagan and Barnett (2003) argue that, when examining the impact of fathers' involvement in the lives of their children, practitioners often disregard the gatekeeping role that mothers in the treatment process take on, which may prevent men from attending. Both the fathers interviewed in the pilot study attended the NVR parenting group with their spouses and we observed that mothers and fathers coming together created opportunities for establishing effective joint parental relationships, which encouraged joint support, and helped rebuild their relationship with their children, which supports the work of Lamb (2004), Boyce *et al* and Howard *et al* (2006).

From our anecdotal experience of running an NVR parenting group with fathers, we found that fathers' involvement can provide much needed support to mothers who are so often left to manage the fallout of challenging young people.

## Tips for encouraging the attendance of fathers

Here are some lessons learned and valuable tips to facilitate the attendance of fathers (including father figures) to NVR groups:

- NVR facilitators would benefit from becoming familiar with the literature and research that highlights the contribution fathers make to their children's lives, allowing them to offer an alternative narrative to the prevailing discourse about mothers' and fathers' roles in child rearing.
- The referral person should include the father or father figure in the recommendations and treatment plan. NVR includes ways to bring parents closer to their children in order to restore their relationships and strengthen parental presence. Fathers often feel isolated and may experience hopelessness

when they see their child misbehaving or displaying a lack of respect towards the parents and the family. The referral person may function as a supporter to the father while he is incorporating different ways of communicating and responding to his child.

- NVR facilitators should become curious if a father is not present or visible at the referral stage of the parenting group.
- Before the NVR group, the father should be interviewed and asked about his views of the situation, and the benefits of the NVR treatment should be explained.
- Allow fathers to express their ambivalence if they are not sure about the NVR programme.
- Invite and allow fathers to share their family's structure, as well as family values and beliefs.
- Increase confidence in fathers' parenting by sharing literature about the importance of their participation.
- Appreciate fathers' participation in the group and follow up their progress.
- At the beginning of each session, ask the group for feedback about the NVR tools that have been practised. Some fathers may struggle to change habits in their parenting, especially if these challenge their own beliefs e.g. de-escalation includes parents not having the last word in a situation (the parent needs to choose to remain quiet or calm, especially if his child escalates).
- Celebrate fathers' small changes and small successes.
- Respond to practical needs by providing interpreters and a crèche as necessary.

# Conclusion

The reasons for fathers' absence in parenting their children is complex. Its foundation is often located in history and in how girls and boys are raised, and this is reinforced by the dominant discourse about social norms and gender roles. The economic workplace, law and polices intersect with this dominant discourse to make women much more visible in child rearing, leaving fathers in the shadows.

That said, we can begin to make new sense of these chronic historic and overlapping external contexts by revisiting our own attitude to fathers. The understanding of fathers' relationships with their children, and with their children's challenging behaviour, needs to be further explored. It is also important to note that the involvement of fathers in their children's treatments and communication with CAMHS and Children's Services needs more exploration through similar studies, and obtaining feedback from each family member.

Effective parent training that includes fathers can achieve a wide range of significant objectives. A clear inference from our study is that professionals need to make extra efforts to include fathers and father figures in the assessment and follow up of their cases, and in suggested interventions and treatments, even in the cases where the father displays resistance or ambivalence.

Parenting training that includes the father has to be the norm. We argue that it is time to move beyond the usual practice of leaving fathers out of treatment plans. Work with adolescents and their families must promote the engagement of fathers. It is time for professionals to think bigger, to commit to making fathers visible in practice and to make fathers and father figures their business. NVR parenting training is one way of engaging and making fathers' presence more visible.

## References

Addis ME & Mahalik JR (2003) Men, masculinity, and the context of seeking help. *American Psychologist* **58** 5–14.

Allen S & Daly K (2007) *The Effects of Father Involvement: An updated research summary of the evidence*. Centre for Families, Work & Well-being. University of Guelph.

Ainsworth MDS, Blehar MC, Waters E & Wall S (1978) *Patterns of Attachment: A psychological study of the strange situation*. New York: Lawrence Erlbaum Associates.

Ball J (2009) Fathering in the shadows: indigenous fathers and Canada's colonial legacies. *The annals of the American Academy* **624** (1) 29–48.

Bee H & Boyd D (2014) *Developing Child*. Essex, England: Pearson Education Ltd.

Boyd-Franklin N & Franklin AJ (2000) *Boys into Men: Raising our African American teenager sons*. New York: Plume Books.

Bowlby J (1982) *Attachment and Loss* (2nd. Ed). New York: Basic Books.

Bowlby J (2005) *A Secure Base: Clinical applications of attachment theory.* London and New York: Routledge Classics.

Bronfenbrenner U (1979) *The Ecology of Human Development: Experiments by nature and design*. Cambridge, MA: Harvard University Press.

Coley RL (2003) Daughter-father relationships and adolescent psychosocial functioning in low- income African American families. *Journal of Marriage and Family* **65** (4) 867–875.

Coley RL & Medeiros BL (2007) Reciprocal longitudinal relations between nonresident father involvement and adolescent delinquency. *Child Development* **78** (1) 132–147.

Cowan CP & PA Cowan (2000) *When Partners Become Parents: The big life change for couples*. Mahwah, NJ: Lawrence Erlbaum.

Day E & Heismann E (2010) *Non-Violent Resistance Programme.* Brighton: Pavilion Publishing & Media Ltd.

 

Dienhart A (2001) Engaging men in family therapy: does the gender of the therapist make a difference? *Journal of Family Therapy* **23** 21–45.

Ellis BJ, Bates JE, Dodge KA, Fergusson DM, Horwood J, Pettit GS & Woodward L (2003) Does father absence place daughters at special risk for early sexual activity and teenage pregnancy? *Child Development* **74** (3) 801–821.

Fagan J & Barnett M (2003) The relationship between maternal gatekeeping, paternal competence, mothers' attitudes about the father role, and father involvement. *Journal of Family Issues* **24** (8) 1020–1043.

Flouri E & Buchanan A (2003) The role of father involvement and mother involvement in adolescents' psychological well-being. *British Journal of Social Work* **33** (3) 399–406.

Field T (1994) The effects of mother's physical and emotional unavailability on emotion regulation. *Monographs of the Society of Research in Child Development* **59** (2-3, Serial No 240).

Field T, Lang C, Yando R & Bendell R (1995) Adolescents' intimacy with parents and friends. *Adolescence* **30** (117) 133–140.

Fernald A (1985) Four-month old infants prefer to listen to mothers. *Infant Behavior and Development* **8** 181–182.

Good GE, Thomson DA & Brathwaite AD (2005) Men and therapy: critical concepts, theoretical frameworks, and research recommendations. *The Journal of Clinical Psychology* **61** 699–711.

Green F (2012) *Practicing Feminist Mothering*. Winnipeg, MB: Arbeiter Ring Publishing.

Griffin KW, Bptvin GJ, Scheier LM, Diaz T & Miller NL (2000) Parenting practices as predictors of substance use, delinquency, and aggression among urban minority youth: Moderating effects of family structure and gender. *Psychology of Addictive Behaviors* **14** (2) 174–184.

Harris KM, Furstenberg FF & Marmer JK (1998) Paternal involvement with adolescents in intact families: the influence of fathers over the life course. *Demography* **35** (2) 201–216.

Heilman B, Levtov R & van der Gaag N, Hassink A & Barker G (2017) *State of the Worlds's Fathers: Time of action*. Washington, DC: Promundo.

Horn WF & Sylvester T (2002) *Father Facts (4th ed)*. National Fatherhood Initiative [online]. Available at: https://www.fatherhood.org/father-absence-statistic (accessed September 2018).

Howard KS, Lefever JE, Borkowski JG & Whitman TL (2006) Fathers' influence in the lives of children with adolescent mothers. *Journal of Family Psychology* **20** (3) 468–476.

Jordan J, McKenna H, Keeney S, Cutcliffe J, Stevenson C, Slater P & McGowan I (2012) Providing Meaningful care: learning from the experience of suicidal young men. *Qualitative Research Health* **22** (9).

Jude J & Rivera-Gould V (2014) Fathers and Non-violent resistance. *Context* **132** 27–28.

Kelly JB (2000) Children's adjustment in conflicted marriage and divorce: A decade review of research. *Journal of the American Academy of child and Adolescent Psychiatry* **39** (8) 963–973.

Krause I & Maitra B (2014) *Culture and Madness*. London: Jessica Kingsley Publishers.

Lamb ME (Ed) (2004) *The Role of the Father in Child Development (4th ed)*. Hoboken, New Jersey: John Wiley & Sons.

Lee CM & Duxbury L (1998) Employed parents' support from partners, employers, and friends. *The Journal of Social Psychology* **138** (3) 303–322.

Milkie M & Peltola P (1999) Playing all the roles: Gender and the work balancing act. *Journal of Marriage and the Family* **61** 476–490.

McLanahan S, Irwin Garfinkel I, Reichman N, Teitler J, Carlson M & Audigier CN (2003) *The fragile families and child well-being study: Baseline National Report*. Princeton, New York: Center for

 

Research on Child Well-being.

O'Reilly A (2008) *Feminist Mothering*. Albany: State University of New York.

Pfiffner LJ, McBurnett K & Rathouz PJ (2001) Father absence and familial antisocial characteristics. *Journal of Abnormal Child Psychology* **29** (5) 357–367.

Richter L & Morrel R (2006) *BABA: Men and Fatherhood in South Africa*. Human Sciences Research Council. Published by HSRC Press.

Rohner RP & Veneziano RA (Eds) (2001) The importance of father love: history and contemporary evidence. *Review of General Psychology* **5** 382-405.

Seltzer J (1991) Relationships between fathers and children who live apart: The father's role after separation. *Journal of Marriage and the Family* **53** (1) 79–101.

Southam-Gerow MA & Philip C, Kendall PC (2000) Emotion regulation and understanding Implications for child psychopathology and therapy. *Clinical Psychology Review* **22** (2002) 189–222.

Thorn GR & Sarata BP (1998) Psychotherapy with African American men: what we know and what we need to know. *Journal of Multicultural Counselling and Development* **26** (4) 240–253.

Van IJzendoorn MH, Juffer F & Duyvesteyn MGC (1995) Breaking the intergenerational cycle of insecure attachment: a review of the effects of attachment-based interventions on maternal sensitivity and infant security. *Journal of Child Psychology and Psychiatry* **36** 225–248.

 

# Chapter 4: Child-focused family therapy using non-violent resistance: hearing the voice of need in the traumatised child

**Dr Peter Jakob**

## Caring dialogue

Adapting NVR can make it a more suitable approach for working with 'trauma-organised systems' (Bentovim, 1995). Jakob (2018) illustrates the larger system aspect of the model I have developed, in which non-violent methods help family members experience greater emotional safety within the wider social environment, enabling the nuclear family to become a recovery environment. This chapter, based on an earlier publication in German (Jakob, 2015), introduces the child-focused aspect of the NVR trauma model.

An integration of child-focused family therapy (Wilson, 1998) with NVR expands the approach to better consider child needs. It centres around the concept of the 'caring dialogue', in which the child expresses distress and an adult shows caring responsiveness, while the child's acceptance of care validates the adult. Certain constraints to such a dialogue appear to be specific to relationships between many children who have been abused and their caregivers. Reconciliation gestures that address unmet needs in the child can re-kindle this dialogue.

Young people who have been abused or neglected often have many unmet psychological needs (D'Andrea *et al*, 2012). Those who develop violent or self-destructive behaviour often reject caregivers and dismiss adults' caring responses (Green & Goldwyn, 2002), and in the process reorganise the social environment: when attempted care is rejected and aggressive behaviour directed at caregivers, how can young people's psychological needs be addressed by the very adults who feel under duress much of the time?

Parental attunement has been identified as a key aspect in the development of secure attachment, which in turn is seen as a major early factor in the trajectory of a person's psycho-social development (e.g. Cozolino, 2014; Wolff & Ijzendoorn, 1997). However, I understand 'attachment' as a reciprocal process – for example, foster carers develop more punitive responses and show fewer caring responses towards children who are dismissive of their care (Dozier *et al*, 2002), corresponding with the clinical observation that caregivers often feel 'erased' when young people show controlling behaviour (Dolberger *et al*, 2016). Carers describe a diminished sense of self, finding it difficult to access internal and interpersonal resources. Considering attachment as a reciprocal process, we cannot use a frame of reference which merely sees the adult as the enabler of secure attachment – we also need to see the child as giving meaning to the adult's responses, validating their sense of self as a caregiver.

> *Relationships between caregivers and children are marked by complex dialogical interaction which enables adults to address child need and promote mutuality. Child distress signals, parental sensitivity to these along with their caring responses, and the child's validation of the adult as caregiver are all constituent parts of this dialogue. Allowing vulnerability requires basic trust, and a child who communicates distress is demonstrating a core belief that the adult is both strong and sensitive to her needs and will not respond in an injurious manner. Caregivers remain attentive and attuned to the child's often hidden or disguised distress signals, and can distinguish between basic psychological needs, wants, and inappropriate demands, and are able to respond in different ways to each of these. They balance protection with support for the child to face developmental challenges, enabling the child to develop their own self-efficacy (Lebowitz & Omer, 2013). Adolescents' distress signals are often ambiguous due to the tension between the need for autonomy and the need for care, so adult support must often find subtle, indirect expression. The child's or adolescent's acceptance of caring responses validates the parent as caregiver, contributing to their self-value and sense of agency. Validation of the parent is further strengthened by non-judgemental discursive practices around the family, which value parental contributions.*

This caring dialogue generates the 'I-Thou relationship' (Buber, 2008): an opening of each self for the experience of the other – here, a genuine encounter between parent and child. A focus on restoring the caring dialogue when constraints have emerged can be therapeutically beneficial, and the aim of child-focused conversations with parents and other caregivers in NVR is to facilitate its re-kindling.

## What happens to adults when young people reject care?

Parental presence is key to non-violent authority (Omer & von Schlippe, 2012). When caregivers who experience rejecting, aggressive or dismissive behaviour avoid the child physically or psychologically by reducing attention, their presence diminishes. Avoidance is a constraint to the child's emotional containment. For example, a mother described 'going off to a far-away island' in her mind whenever her son entered the room, to avoid being flooded by fear and humiliation. His mother's dissociative response became a constraint to perceiving any distress signals he may have communicated.

Parents with histories of interpersonal abuse can develop pronounced avoidance behaviours. The child's physical presence alone can become associated in the parent's mind with earlier trauma: 'When he gets that look in his eyes, I see his dad, it makes my hair stand on end…'. This leaves the adult feeling threatened and experiencing fear, rage, humiliation, shame or victim guilt. Such survival reactivity can activate intense avoidance; alternatively, traumatised parents may show a fight response, hypo-arousal, or experience intrusive memories.

Some parents become preoccupied with physical or emotional injury by their child, wishing to 'show him how it feels'. Negative internal representations of one another in conflictual relationships are associated with reduced empathy (Grace *et al*, 1993). Neuro-psychological studies demonstrate that the impulse for revenge is associated with a lowering of activity in brain regions which are generally activated when an individual feels empathy (see Pinker, 2011, p577).

Hughes and Baylin (2012) describe caring responses such as being sensitive and emotionally responsive, comforting children effectively and consistently, enabling them to learn how to enjoy and stay connected to other people, knowing when children struggle and helping them build resilience, and protecting children from the dysregulating effects of adults' own negative emotions by being self-regulated. Their concept of 'blocked care' describes an inability to perform the above functions, and suggests a therapeutic focus on the parent's own past experiences, 'in order to defuse negative potential for unresolved painful memories to disrupt their parenting and their child's development' (p41).

However, understandings of 'blocked care' can, in my experience, feed into victim-blaming discourses, leaving parents feeling guilty and ashamed. Feeling blamed is a key problem for parents in adolescent-to-parent violence (Holt, 2013). The concept of the 'caring dialogue' offers a constraint model derived from Narrative Therapy (White & Epston, 1990) as an alternative to the potentially pathologising premise of an *inability to care*. It sees parents as potentially able to actualise internal and inter-personal resources and follows the understanding in Solution Focused Therapy that solution contexts differ from the causational contexts of problems (de Shazer, 1988). Certain constraints may mitigate against the parent's potential for caring interaction, and against validation of parents in their caring role, but these factors do not have to render the caring dialogue impossible in the here and now.

In my view, interaction around care may emerge *quickly* between parent and child, if at least one party – the parents – can be supported to *imagine* a dialogical exchange around their child's needs and can be supported to perform acts of care in certain significant instances. Imagining care and practising caring acts can then weaken the impact of the constraints.

## How do young people with harmful behaviour deal with distress?

Adolescents with behavioural problems have more highly activated amygdala function than others (Herpertz *et al*, 2008; Ohman, 2005), and this hyper-arousal is associated with exaggerated perception of risk within the social environment (Vasterling & Brewin, 2005). Young people who act aggressively live in a subjectively threatening world, experiencing 'the other' as intrinsically hostile (Barrett *et al*, 1996). A young person who experiences adults as hostile is unlikely to seek solace or support from them.

Moments of expressed need – a very brief signalling of distress by the young person – can be instantly followed by aggressive responses. In these cases the young person appears to have grown accustomed to displacing a vulnerable state of mind with angry aggression. Mentalisation may be constrained; instead of, 'I'm feeling troubled, confused, I'm scared,' we hear, 'You piss me off, I wish you were dead!' When anger immediately displaces distress, the child cannot 'hear their own voice of distress'.

Young people with histories of maltreatment may show controlling behaviour in order to increase the predictability of their environment, and the child's needs become difficult to address. The rapidly growing mutual alienation can result in the child feeling alone, unwanted and with a diminished sense of belonging.

 

A vicious cycle emerges as the young person becomes ever more unlikely to sustain any feeling of vulnerability.

Young people with controlling behaviour often complain they 'never get anything', that their caregivers 'don't want them to have anything' – in spite of the attention or material things they often demand and receive. There seems to be a problematic relational logic at work: persistently controlling behaviour curtails sufficient experience of *receiving without antecedent demand.* A child who persistently takes will have little opportunity to *receive*, and it can be very difficult for caregivers to find the opportunity to *give* rather than *have taken* from them; yet *receiving* is necessary for the experience of unconditional love and acceptance, which a young person with a history of maltreatment often desperately needs.

## Unconditional love and care: I will always reach out to you, regardless of what you do...

How can systemic work with NVR address child needs, if the clinician works generally with adults? Hermans speaks of a 'polyphonic self' (2001). The 'self' can be seen as having a multiplicity of positions, which depend on the positions of the other(s); there is no core self. Omer (2004) uses the metaphor of the 'orchestra of voices', positing 'positive' yet unheard 'voices' in the aggressive child: the child has positive attributes, needs love and guidance, and can become more self-regulated, when the parent's strength increases. These positions are seen as being already potentially inherent in the person of the child, and Omer posits that adults can address such 'positive' yet 'unheard voices' by avoiding any escalatory response while challenging child aggression, and by persistently showing the child their love and acceptance through the performance of reconciliation gestures (further referred to as 'relational reconciliation gestures').

Wilson (1998) also uses the 'voice' metaphor: the voice of need has become silent. A child focus is achieved by speaking *with*, not *at* the child. In this way, a narrative can emerge that associates new meaning with child behaviour (Jakob *et al*, 2014) and may enable the adults to perceive distress even when it has been obscured by the veil of harmful and destructive behaviour.

I have integrated principles of Wilson's child-focused family therapy into NVR (Jakob, 2011). Speaking *with* a child to gain insight into their distress opens a dialogical process, but one must get there first: helping adult and child find their way (back) to a genuine encounter with one another becomes an aim of therapeutic conversation. I concur with Wilson (2012) that a child focus does not equate to adopting a child-centred position; if therapist and parents or other caregivers acted in a child-centred way against the immediate backdrop of harmful behaviour, they would inadvertently privilege the 'loud voice of aggression'.

The parent may first need to experience strength by taking positive action against harmful behaviour, if we are to open space for attention and attunement to the child, so that they no longer respond from a position of erasure or survival reactivity. Once the child is perceived as having need they are no longer seen as a threatening antagonist, but the parent's perception of the child expressing need will initially need to be largely imaginary. Perceiving 'the other' as a fellow human being who can suffer and has needs lies at the heart of socio-political non-violent resistance, as conceptualised and practiced by Gandhi, Martin Luther King and others (Rappoport, 1990). Humanising 'the other' becomes a leap of faith.

Yet how can the adult enter a dialogue when the child shows no apparent willingness to engage in it? The principle of one-sided action (Lebowitz & Omer, 2013), which allows determined resistance against destructive behaviour, can also enable adults to persistently invite children into dialogue. The therapist first assists parents in planning and imagining an act of resistance they will undertake in response to recent problematic behaviour, enabling *a moment of strength*. Parents can then carefully plan and persistently implement relational reconciliation gestures, *regardless* of whether the young person shows a positive response to their efforts or not. This requires them to become able to *internally* relate to the 'voice of need' in the child and imagine that the child is *potentially* capable of expressing this voice. Only if relational gestures are made without any expectation that the young person will show immediate appreciation do they become acts of unconditional love and acceptance. Persistent but not insistent unsolicited parental acts of care enable the young person to experience attention they have not demanded. Precisely because a parent persists in showing care in the face of rejection, they can establish a new relational logic; the message is: 'You do not need to take – you receive, without needing to force me'. Hardly a message can be more powerful than that of persistent goodwill in the face of rejection – the child eventually realises that the parent must 'really mean it' and over time may develop a felt sense of the adult's unconditionality.

The therapeutic vehicle for such parental sensitisation to particular 'unheard voices' is planning relational gestures that draw parental attention from their own emotional injury towards their child's needs. When parents see themselves responding with care to distress signals, and imagine their child validating them by accepting such care, the adult's compassionate responsiveness can become reactivated, even if the child is not yet reciprocating in the here and now. Persistently carrying out relational, need-related reconciliation gestures then gives the child the message, that the adult will not be deterred from care by aggression or rejection. The implicit message is: '*No matter how often you reject us – we are your parents (carers), you cannot shake off our care!*'

## Unmet needs

The categories below have emerged from my work with traumatised children, and can act as a guide to help parents sensitise themselves to child need.

**The need for safety.** Many children and young people with histories of child maltreatment show post-traumatic responsiveness, as well as signs of insecurity in their attachment to adult caregivers, which has been conceptualised as a specific form of post-traumatic stress (Hansen & Spratt, 2000) in which the basic trust in the continuity of care by the other person has been undermined and which results in interpersonal anxiety relating to closeness and intimacy. Growing mutual trust is necessary if the family (or home) is to become a 'recovery environment' (Jakob, 2018) for trauma. The child's unmet need here is for developing a felt sense of safety and protection in the adult's presence.

**The need for control of one's life: accomplishment.** In self-determination theory, 'autonomous motivation' in the pursuit of goal-directed action is seen as a central motivation (Koestner *et al*, 2008). This need to feel in control of one's own life while experiencing the intrinsic ability and competency to do so can be seen, more simply, as the need for a sense of accomplishment. I often find that attention to supporting a sense of accomplishment in both academic achievement and social competence is a key component of successful therapeutic outcomes for traumatised children.

Families are prone to experiencing crises at significant transitional stages within the life cycle (Carter & McGoldrick, 1999; Carr, 2006). It is reasonable to assume that developmental difficulties, such as attachment insecurity, being on the autism spectrum or having learning difficulties, can further exacerbate stress upon the family at such transitional stages. When adults reinstate themselves as supporters to a child's accomplishment, this can become a key factor in the family's and the child's recovery, as well as in the positive atmosphere and functioning of the classroom.

**The need to feel a sense of belonging.** Not feeling they belong is a common complaint of young people who show aggressive behaviour and have become disaffected in relationships with their caregivers. Children and adolescents in foster or residential care struggle significantly in this regard, and the repeated breakdown of care arrangements exacerbates their sense of isolation. Reconciliation gestures representing inclusion address this need.

**The need for a coherent and benign narrative of self and family.** Children who have experienced abuse tend to construct narratives of interpersonal relationships which are incoherent in structure and threatening in content, and much more fragmented than others (Hodges & Steele, 2000). However, adults who can tell coherent stories of their own traumatic childhoods are likely to have securely attached children themselves (Steele *et al*, 2003; Byng-Hall, 1997), indicating that a coherent family or attachment narrative may be beneficial. Vetere and Dallos (2009; Dallos, 2004) have developed a systemic/attachment-focused perspective which promotes children's ability to perceive and utilise other people as a coping resource when they feel threatened. They consider a coherent 'attachment narrative' in which significant others are represented in a sufficiently positive way to be a therapeutic vehicle for increasing attachment security.

## Rekindling the caring dialogue

Change can be effectively instigated when therapist and client find small, pivotal actions that feel profoundly meaningful to family members, and which are likely to have a significant impact on patterns of interaction within the family. These can be child-focused relational reconciliation gestures, and their planning enables parental (re)sensitisation to unmet needs. Taking one-sided action by carrying out these gestures persistently and regardless of the young person's rejection or dismissal, becomes a standing invitation for them to trust caregivers, eventually promoting the young person's awareness of the adult's sensitivity to their needs, and suggesting they could show vulnerability rather than aggression. The therapist's task is merely to help facilitate the rekindling of the caring dialogue by supporting the parent to plan and carry out their gestures.

## Imagery of dialogue

Imagery of caring dialogue can 'thicken the plot', creating narratives of successful future interaction, which run counter to the earlier pervasive victim narratives. These preferred futures are further stimulated by visualising relational reconciliation gestures the parent would like to make. In this way, the repair of relational rupture in the parent's mind can precede the repair of relational rupture in actual interaction. Such a process is intuitive and embodied, and very different from 'trauma speculation', which often objectifies young people in the guise of empathy. I will briefly introduce two out of an array of methods I use with caregivers to help re-kindle the caring dialogue:

 

## The imaginary caring conversation

Before engaging with their own imagery, it is important that the parent can experience a moment of strength, either by remembering positive action they have taken against the child's controlling behaviour in the past or by planning future positive action. The parent is then invited to imagine that a situation might occur in the future with *even less volatile behaviour,* in which the child would signal distress more clearly, and the parent would communicate their compassion. Parent and therapist share their imagery in a collaborative generative process, co-creating the story of a caring dialogue that is yet to come. The adult can imagine being attentive and attuned to the child, verbally or non-verbally encouraging the child to confide in them without intrusion or insistence, and thereby develop a felt sense of what it will be like to raise her caring presence, while mindfully allowing enough distance for the child to be able to cope with their own sense of vulnerability.

Here is an example of the therapist's verbalisations in an 'imaginary caring conversation'.

> *'So, you've decided to do a sit-in for when he kicked his sister after school yesterday. Once you've done that, can you imagine, one day, Jack comes home from school, and he's angry – just not as aggressive as usual?'*
>
> *'OK, so he goes up to his room. Maybe you make him a cup of tea – can you see yourself bringing it up to him? Perhaps you're standing outside his half open door and looking in – what do you see?'*
>
> *'So, you see him lying on the bed, facing the wall. OK, so you're putting the cup of tea down next to him. You're quietly sitting there. I wonder, after a little while, what do you say?'*
>
> *'OK, so you're saying, "Bad day at school, huh?" What is he doing? What does he say?'*
>
> *'So, let's ask him now, what small gesture you can make that will remind him you get it, so he can feel understood, but doesn't have to talk about it too much, so he can save face?'*
>
> *'So, he's shrugging his shoulders, but it feels like he'd like a gesture – oh, so he's saying just a text from you when he's at school…'*
>
> *'OK, so when you start sending texts in real life, what will help you avoid the trap of expecting a positive response from him? So that you don't react with disappointment, or anger, or feel discouraged, if he doesn't respond positively?'*

In the following session, therapist and parent can discuss what the parent has experienced once she has actually carried out the needs-based relational gesture.

## Interviewing the 'internalised child-in-need'

Interviewing the 'internalised other' (Mundry *et al*, 2016) aims to help facilitate empathy. I use the internalised other interview in child-focused NVR to support parents to 'reach behind the veil' of the child's problematic communication in their own imagination. This can help them develop a felt sense of how the young person *may in the future* communicate distress and express their unmet needs. The therapist speaks to the parent as if they were their own child, asking the 'child' questions about their needs, and how their 'parents' could respond to these needs. This privileging of the unheard voice of need in the child aims to almost literally make it audible – with the parent's voice becoming the surrogate voice for their child.

Throughout such imaginary processes, it can be useful for the therapist to keep the aforementioned areas of unmet need in traumatised children in mind, in order to help elicit a wide scope of parental empathy for the child. The NVR principle of persistence seems to be key to a positive impact on the actual parent/child relationship: rather than expecting an appreciative response, caregivers are encouraged to repeatedly make needs-based reconciliation gestures without insisting on validation or appreciation, instead remaining internally connected with their images of the child-as-potentially-able-to-express-their-distress. While there is no comparative outcome research to date, my own therapeutic experience appears to indicate a significant speeding up of the NVR process through this generative process.

When children have been harmed by a parent in the past, imaginary caring dialogue can further support the parent to acknowledge and take responsibility for their own past behaviour. By explicitly taking responsibility and showing empathy for the hurt the child has experienced, the parent communicates to the child that they respect their integrity and sees them as worthy of protection. This carefully prepared gesture of reconciliation – usually as a formal letter that the parent reads out loud to their child – becomes a key reconnective act of reparation for some of the most severe relational ruptures between parent and child, and can act as the beginning of further dialogue.

## Reflections

There is a rich reservoir of methods in family therapy, such as therapeutic metaphors and family rituals, with which therapists can support parents to creatively construct needs-based relational reconciliation gestures that aim to restore the parent/child relationship, and thereby contribute to the family or home becoming a more effective recovery environment for the young person. However, practitioners may attempt to promote parental sensitivity to the child but neglect the need to facilitate parental strength in the resistance against harmful or self-destructive behaviour. Only a parent feeling strong and resourceful can empathise and care. In the both/and of strength-building resistance and care-orientated reconciliation lies the essence of child-focused NVR.

## References

Bentovim A (1995) *Trauma-organized systems: physical and sexual abuse in families*. London: Karnac.

Byng-Hall J (1997) Toward a coherent story in illness and loss. In: R. Papadopoulos and J. Byng-Hall (eds.) *Multiple Voices: Narratives in sys temic family psychotherapy*. London: Duckworth.

Barrett PM, Rapee RM, Dadds MM & Ryan SM (1996) Family enhancement of cognitive style in anxious and aggressive children. *Journal of Abnormal Child Psychology* **24** (2) pp87–203.

Buber M (2013) *I and thou* (2nd ed). London: Continuum.

Carr A (2006) *The handbook of child and adolescent clinical psychology.* London: Routledge.

Carter B & McGoldrick M (1999) The expanded family lifecycle. *Individual family and social perspectives* (3rd ed). Boston: Allyn & Bacon.

Cozolino L (2014) *The Neuroscience of Human Relationships: Attachment and the developing social brain* (Norton Series on Interpersonal Neurobiology). NY: Norton.

Dallos R (2004) Attachment narrative therapy: integrating ideas from narrative and attachment theory in systemic family therapy with eating disorders. *Journal of Family Therapy* **26** (1) pp40–65.

D'Andrea W, Ford J, Stolbach B, Spinazzola J & Van der Kolk BA (2012) Understanding interpersonal trauma in children: why we need a developmentally appropriate trauma diagnosis. *American Journal of Orthopsychiatry* **82** (2) pp187–200.

De Shazer S (1988) *Clues: Investigating solutions in Brief Therapy*. New York: W.W. Norton.

Dolberger D, Fried M & Jakob P (2016) The presence mind: functional states of consciousness and responsiveness. *Presentation at the 4th International Conference on Non-Violent-Resistance, Malmoe, Sweden*, 26th-27th May.

Dozier M, Higley E, Albus KE & Nutter A (2002) Interviewing with foster infants' caregivers: targeting three critical needs. *Infant Mental Health Journal* **23** (5) pp541–554.

Grace NC, Kelley ML & McCain AP (1993) Attribution processes in mother-adolescent conflict. *Journal of Abnormal Child Psychology* **21** (2) pp199–211.

Green J & Goldwyn R (2002) Annotation; attachment disorganisation and psychopathology: new findings in attachment research and their potential implications for developmental psychopathology in childhood. *The Journal of Child Psychology and Psychiatry* **43** (7) pp835–846.

Hansen RF & Spratt EG (2000) Reactive attachment disorder: what we know about the disorder and implications for treatment. *Child Maltreatment* **5** (2) pp137–145.

Hermans HJM (2001) The dialogical self: towards a theory of personal and cultural positioning. *Culture and Psychology* **7** (3) pp323–365.

Herpertz SC, Huebner T, Marx I, Vloet TD, Fink GR, Stoecker T, Shah NJ, Konrad K & Herpertz-Dahlmann B (2008) Boys with early onset conduct disorders hyperarousal of the amygdala: emotional processing in male adolescents with childhood onset conduct disorder. *Journal of Child Psychology and Psychiatry* **49** (7) pp781–791.

Hodges J & Steele M (2000) Effects of abuse on attachment representations: narrative assessments of abused children. *Journal of Child Psychotherapy* **26** (3) pp433–455.

Holt A (2013) *Adolescent to Parent Abuse: Current understandings in research, policy and practice*. Bristol: Policy Press.

Hughes DA & Baylin J (2012) *Brain-based Parenting: The neuroscience of caregiving for healthy attachment*. New York, London: W.W. Norton.

Jakob P (2015) Child-focused family therapy using Non Violent Resistance. The voice of need in the aggressive child – from relational reconciliation gestures to restoring parental sensitivity. *Familiendynamik* **40** (1) pp46–55.

Jakob P (2011) *Reconnecting parents and young people with serious behaviour problems – childfocused practice and reconciliation work in Non Violent Resistance Therapy. Tel Aviv: New Authority Network International* [online]. Available at: http://www.newauthority.net/data/cntfiles/146_.pdf (accessed September 2018).

Jakob P (2018) Multi-stressed families, child violence and the larger system: an adaptation of the nonviolent model. *Journal of Family Therapy* **40** 25–44.

Jakob P, Wilson J & Newman M (2014) Non-violence and a focus on the child: a UK perspective. *Context* **132** (2) 37–41.

Koestner R, Otis N, Powers TA, Pelletier L & Gagnon H (2008) Autonomous motivation, controlled motivation, and goal progress. *Journal of Personality* **76** (5) pp1201–1229.

Lebowitz E & Omer H (2013) *Treating Childhood and Adolescent Anxiety: A guide for caregivers*. Hoboken: Wiley.

Mundry TE, Strong T, Sametband I, Rogers-de Jong M, Gaete J, Merritt S, Doyle EM & Ross KH (2016) Internalized other interviewing in relational therapy: three discursive approaches to understanding its use and outcomes. *Journal of Marital and Family Therapy* **42** (1) 168–184.

Ohmann A (2005) The role of the amygdala in human fear: automatic detection of threat. *Psychoneuroendocrinology* **30** (10) pp953–958.

Omer H (2004) *Nonviolent Resistance: A new approach to violent and selfdestructive children*. Cambridge: Cambridge University Press.

Omer H & von Schlippe A (2012) *Authority without violence: Coaching for parents of children with behavioural problems*. Göttingen: Vandenhoeck & Ruprecht.

Pinker S (2011) *The Better Angels of Our Nature: The decline of violence in history and its causes*. London: Penguin.

Rappoport L (1990) Power, personality and the dialectics of nonviolence. In: VK Kool (ed) *Perspectives on Nonviolence*. New York: Springer.

Steele M, Steele H, Wooger M, Yabsley S, Fonagy P, Johnson D & Croft C (2003) An attachment perspective on children's emotion narratives: links across generations. In: RN Embe, DP Wolf & D Oppenheim (eds.) *Revealing the Inner Worlds of Young Children: The MacArthur story stem battery and parent – child narratives*. Oxford: Oxford University Press.

Vasterling JJ & Brewin C (2005) *Neuropsychology of PTSD*. New York: Guilford Press.

Vetere A & Dallos R (2008) Systemic therapy and attachment narratives. *Journal of Family Therapy* **30** (4) pp374–385.

 

White M & Epston D (1990) *Narrative Means to Therapeutic Ends*. New York: W.W. Norton.

Wilson J (2012) *Personal communication*.

Wilson J (1998) *Childfocused Practice: A collaborative systemic approach.* London: Karnac.

Wolff MS & Ijzendoorn MH (1997) Sensitivity and attachment: a meta-analysis on parental antecedents of infant attachment. *Child Development* **68** (4) pp571–591.

# Chapter 5: Coaching, safeguarding and NVR – supporting parents to keep their children safe

**By Julia Jude with Sarah Blyth**

## Introduction

The issue of safeguarding children from trafficking, gangs, peer-on-peer violence, sexual exploitation, cyber pornography, sexual predation, radicalisation and extremism has become a focus of concern in the new wave of social work practice (Wood, 2016; Condry & Miles 2012; NSPCC, 2014; Pona *et al*, 2015). As a result, governments are looking for creative and innovative ways of working directly with issues of safeguarding to support children and their families (Forrester *et al*, 2013; Goodman & Trowler, 2012; Munro, 2011). However, Firmin (2017) argues that the current framework used to safeguard young people has its limitations as it does not recognise the relevance of extra-familial contexts that put young people at risk, undermine parental capacity and professionals' ability to safeguard young people.

In this chapter, we argue that the principles of NVR offer a creative and innovative framework for coaching parents so they might better develop their safeguarding skills and improve their parental capacity to respond to wider situations that threaten and undermine adolescent and parenting relationships and which often lead to child parent abuse (Newman *et al,* 2014).

The need to do something different within the context of safeguarding is echoed by Wood (2016), Munro *et al* (2016) and Munro (2011), who argue that there is a need for practitioners to move towards using a range of approaches to safeguarding, including practice-based interventions. Preston-Shoot (2017) suggests that attention should be directed to having a systemic overview of the problems associated with safeguarding, which would explore the inherently complex contexts which safeguarding operates in that produce fractured and fragmented practice.

Firmin (2017) argues that safeguarding assessments are much too narrow, focusing on individualised family systems and background data which she notes are largely desk-based exercises informed by assessments, intervention plans, reports and minutes etc. She observed that much more attention needs to be given to extra-familial contexts such as bullying in school, victimisation on public transport, anti-social behaviour and criminality, contexts where young people are at risk in public spaces.

There are two threads that connects Munro (2011), Preston–Shoot (2017) and Firmin, 2017. First, that a systemic approach to safeguarding is needed to address the limitations of legislation put in place to safeguard young people. Second, that to meet the needs of families faced with the challenging complexity of safeguarding requires re-imagining and creating approaches that can respond to the situated and often complex local contexts that face children and families in times of need.

## Why we need a different response for safeguarding practice?

Creating new ways of supporting families in times of need requires some consideration of how we intervene, and how parents access services (Dalzell & Sawyer, 2016). Condry and Miles (2012; 2013) claim that there is little assistance for parents and, additionally, mainstream services are often ill-equipped to support them.

Coogan (2012) and Omer (2004; 2011) claim that children who find themselves faced with safeguarding issues often tend to be emotionally, physically and verbally challenging in their home. Moreover, these challenging behaviours tend to result in child parent abuse in many families that goes beyond cultures. This view fits with Coogan's (2012) observations that adults who lack strong parenting skills, or who have issues which affect their ability to parent, are more likely to be victims of abuse, and in some cases these conflicts can escalate to the point that parents may feel redundant and fearful of setting boundaries for their child (Weinblatt & Omer, 2008). According to Ford (2015) the helplessness of some parents has resulted in parents turning to the Metropolitan Police to keep the peace at home and in the community. Condry and Miles (2013) agree that parents are turning to police but claim that this occurs as a result of services failing families and children. Firmin's (2017) study, meanwhile, illuminated that professionals are struggling with how best to work with the challenges of extra-familial risk that young people face and that undermines parental capacity. Firmin (2017) further suggests that a systemic methodology in safeguarding could offer a contextual lens that shifts the clinical gaze from gathering data from textual contexts to gathering data from the lived experiences of the young people and the specific situated contexts where self-harming responses emerge.

## Skills development requires practice

The conversations and debates regarding safeguarding are not new and will continue, often triggered by serious case reviews (Preston-Shoot, 2017; Wood, 2016; Laming, 2003). Firmin (2017) and Preston-Shoot (2017) offer tangible pathways for re-thinking safeguarding practices and agree with Munro *et al* (2016) that deliberation – a process of focus thinking – has an important role to play in safeguarding.

Systemic ideas that privilege deliberation through the process of self and relational reflexivity could further enhance practices that invite awareness and understanding as well as doing and performing one's understanding. As noted by Preston-Shoot (2017) safeguarding is a complicated entanglement of relational and complex responses which requires practitioners and agencies to work more collaboratively with parents, as now safeguarding is a concern which goes beyond the walls of the family home and has spilled into the community and beyond (Condry & Miles, 2013).

However, Firmin (2017) argues that parental capacity is not where the focus should be and suggests that additional attention should be directed to the situated specific contexts where extra-familial activity is occurring. We argue that extra-familial contexts need to be considered alongside support that helps parents to develop and sustain parental capacity. NVR approaches have supported parents to respond to extra-familial contexts; The Parent Patrol is one example, in which parents volunteer to tour their locality and engage with young people who are out and about, making their presence visible as a way of reducing dangerous behaviour (Gilad, 2017).

Supporting parents to develop their capacity to safeguard their children who encounter extra-familial contexts which lead to parent abuse requires an element of coaching. We argue that following the critical moment that brought outside services into the family home, NVR can provide a framework for continued safeguarding. In this model, parents and carers should be equipped with the skills to work with their sons and daughters, fostered and adopted young people, long after the professionals have ceased their involvement. The practice framework of NVR offers parents skills and knowledge as a way of keeping their children safe within their community. These practical abilities emerge through teaching the principles of NVR that focus on establishing relational responses. These relational abilities could be described as a set of constitutive rules (Searle, 1969) informed by specific tasks, activities, routines and actions which parents are encouraged to perform within the training context and in their own homes. By giving parents skills they become stronger and feel less helpless and better able to safeguard their children (Omer, 2011; Day & Heismann, 2010).

## NVR coaching: learning from doing

Schatzki *et al* (2001), Merleau-Ponty (1983) and Todes (2007) claim that the acquiring of skills involves practice. They suggest that it is through action and interaction (doing, telling and performing) that knowledge emerges and social life is organised, reproduced and transformed. In support of the above scholarly claims, Bateson (2016) argues that language and words in themselves are empty and that 'words are delicious, but cannot say much… they often lose the water of meaning before it is delivered… There is no language to define the spiralling processes of the vast context we are participants in' (p3).

These ideas are not new and so you might wonder why they need stating. There is evidence that our mainstream psychological theories are married to the Cartesian view (Shotter, 2016; Feyerabend,1987) that knowledge and meaning-making happen through cognitive processes in the individual's mind. As a result, these ideas privilege theory over practice and dismiss the body and environment in the role of the acquisition of knowledge. And while we do not disagree that theory has a place in knowledge formation, we would add that experience of doing is pivotal to acquiring skills as noted by Schatzki *et al* (2001).

Higashia (2017), a young man who talks of his experience of living with autism, noted that theory, dialogue and visual cues could not replace the importance of doing, experience and observation, which he claims is where his learning stems from. We argue that a safeguarding framework could be organised around the idea of coaching; a process that supports learning and development by way of role play and through the process of experimenting with different ways of doing (Gallwey, 1986). Borrowing from Gallwey, we argue that NVR provides a valuable coaching structure that embraces a body of activities built on a practical understanding that emerges within the approach. Principally, NVR embeds the idea of learning from doing, learning from the service user's own experience, learning that appreciates and encourages feedback from others and listening to the feedback of others.

Parents are encouraged, assisted, inspired and nurtured to become aware of their responses and abilities as a way of enhancing their ability to notice improvements in their relationships with their children. Within that context, the performance of NVR principles is significant: it is not generalised but subjectively and intimately related to the parents' experience, which is context specific (Dewey, 1934).

According to Merleau-Ponty (1983), Searle (1969) and Wittgenstein (1953), we learn through doing and through action. These philosophers argue that dialogue and theory is no substitute for practice. Within the framework of NVR, this gets translated into parents being encouraged to work with the idea of making and performing their relationship and being attentive to what gets created. In the doing of relationships, parents become aware of the skills involved in the relational responses that emerge between self and others. What is being attempted is a process whereby parents are encouraged to make visible the physical presence of their actions/responses. This creates opportunities for parents to become relationally reflexive and aware of their roles and responsibilities (Gergen, 2009; Etherington, 2007).

What follows is an account by Sarah Blyth (co-author) of her experience of NVR as a coaching framework, using the method of autoethnography to share and explore her personal account and the understanding that emerged from her experience.

## Case example

Gangs work in a clever way; they notice when an adolescent is having a bad time at home, and when the parent and adolescent relationship has broken down. Gang members often groom the adolescent to make them feel important and special. Giving the adolescent a feeling of self-worth and belonging as the adolescent sees the gang as a substitute for their family, which gives gang members the leverage to gain control over the adolescent, creating a pathway of separation and distance between them and their parents. This leaves the parents feeling that they have lost the young person to the gang, as their loyalty lies within the gang membership. This is what happened to my family, and to my son.

Before doing the NVR parent group, our house was a living hell. Every day there would be violence, abusive language and holes being punched in walls, and physical and mental abuse was a daily occurrence. As a parent I had no control.

I could not protect my daughter or myself from my son. I spent my days crying and feeling low. My confidence had gone, my love for my son had been knocked out of me physically, I hated my son and I was afraid of him.

I felt alone and isolated and too ashamed to tell others what life at home was like. So I pretended – I put on a smile and tried to get through one violent day at a time.

I heard of an NVR parent group from our social worker but I didn't have much faith in NVR as I had done other parenting groups and they didn't help – we just spent a lot of time talking and then when I got home the situation was still the same. We had also been referred to family therapy sessions, which did not work as my son would sit and listen to what I had said to the therapist and would use what he had heard against me.

I decided to give NVR a try as I was desperate. I was shocked to see how many other parents were going through the same nightmare as myself. It was good not to feel judged when I told the group of my experience. And it was a relief to unload to a group of people who had similar experiences as myself. I no longer had to hide but could just say what was going on for me at home. The NVR group was my freedom from the violence that I was being subjected to; it gave me time for me.

I found the NVR tools really effective when put into practice at home. For example, the announcement helped me to regain my confidence as a parent. I remember using the words, 'I will no longer tolerate'. This felt that I was finally making a stand as a parent. It felt good, as I was able to believe in myself again as a parent.

But it was not all plain sailing. The self-announcement was an activity that I found very emotional. It made me take a good look at my inner self. And there I encountered where I may have been at fault with my parenting which, over the years, had contributed to making my son's behaviour controlling.

During the NVR parenting group, we practised the NVR tools through role play. This was very powerful as I could get a feel of how my son might react as I attempted to put the NVR tool into practice. Through the coaching, I learnt not to judge or put blame on my son. I became aware of the importance of choosing the right wording so I would make a connection with my son before correction. I would make sure my timing was right, this way there was no blame and the situation didn't escalate into my son becoming violent towards me.

When my son was out and didn't answer his phone, I would look for his friends' telephone numbers and call their phones or leave a text. By doing this I was making my parental presence known to the gang members. (My son soon would answer his phone the next time I rang him.)

I'd tidy my son's bedroom to show my parental presence – if I came across any drugs I would keep hold of them. By doing this my son knew I'd found them. And I was aware of his activities on the street. By holding onto the drugs I'd found, I was actively acting on the situation, my son knew the only way he would find out where the drugs were would be by asking me. To resist escalation, when my son asked where the drugs were and if I could give them back to him, in a calm but firm voice I would say, 'I do not want to see them brought back into our house again'. (As a parent I wanted to flush the drugs down the toilet, but I knew I couldn't as this would put my son in great danger with the gang members.) By doing the role play and coaching I felt more confident and able to transfer the idea from the group context into our home.

Before the NVR, I was involved with the police, anger management sessions, social services, family therapy, school counsellors, was on the at risk register and threatened with eviction from our home. I'm glad to say that we are no longer in need of these services.

And so where are we as a family today? Well, my son is no longer evolved in the gang, he has really turned his life around. He has been working for eight months on a building site, which he really enjoys. I am so proud of him, and I'm glad I didn't give up on him through the troublesome times.

How can we describe the transformation and movement that Sarah described? Drawing on Merleau-Ponty (1983) Searle (1969) and Wittgenstein's (1953) ideas of learning through doing and rule-making, it could be argued that Sarah is describing a period in her family life during which there was a lack of order and rules that meant she was unable to confidently speak with authority, which led to the derailment of her ability to parent. Wittgenstein (1953) and Searle (1969) argue that we need concrete structures/rules to manage our day-to-day existence. It could be argued that Sarah was performing being a parent but did not have an anchor (rules) to support her role.

Sarah notes that she had tried other services, which provided insight and encouraged her to think about her situation. But Wittgenstein (1953) and Shotter (2016) argue that thinking is not the same as doing, and that acting into a situation allows you to be intimately acquainted with the context – a view point supported by Higashida (2017). Sarah observed that in the role plays she was able to practise new skills in the group, which she found helpful. Wittgenstein, (1953), Shotter (2016) and Higashia (2017) suggest that insight and cognitive information is not helpful in developing practice. They maintain that what is required is practice, routine, experience and habit. According Schatzki, Cetina and Savigny (2001), when you take part in practice (as Sarah did in the group) you enter a space that offers a level of acquaintance to the issue in focus, you develop expectations, you receive direct feedback and respond to the relational context that you are in with the others. From Sarah's narrative, she shifted from not knowing how to go on with the difficulties experienced to becoming aware, which, Wittgenstein (1953) argues, is a shift from blindness to awareness.

But it was not all plain sailing. Sarah mentions the wave of emotions she felt during the announcement, which I refer to as 'reflexivity of discomfort' (Pillow,

2003) that speaks to the vulnerability of the individual. The application of reflexivity of discomfort is an awareness that parents and adolescents are exposed to many contexts that create conditions that make their relationship vulnerable to both external and internal flux and to the actions of self and others. Reflexivity of discomfort is an important concept in bringing forth change, and critical for the rebuilding of relationships. This is based on the idea that parents will get in touch with vulnerable points within the self during the course of the programme which creates a shift from power over the other to having power with the other (Starhawk, 1987). Sarah's example provided many moments where the coaching intervention led to having power, rather than having power over her son.

The framework below offers a lens through which we might make sense of the process involved in using coaching as a safeguarding approach to practice. The framework includes:

- **Acceptance** of the situation and circumstances that the parent has found him/herself in. This encourages a shift from what is going on in the mind of the parent and invites instead an appreciation of the practice by exploring what happens in a moment and exploring through action. This was illuminated in Sarah's example where she made reference to her role/responsibility and previous family context that might have contributed to aspects of her son's controlling behaviour.
- **Connecting** with expectations, beliefs/values, emotions and the consequences of certain actions which includes the core values that underpin ideas around parenting. The emphasis on values differs from traditional theories on parenting as it goes beyond intellectual linguistic accounts of dialoguing of values into a bodily and performative experience of otherness (Levinas, 2006). The process of showing how speech acts are performed is a powerful way of understanding and making sense of how our responses impact on ourselves and others. Again, Sarah's example of reading out her announcement in the group gave her opportunities to become mindful of her breathing, the pacing of her utterance, the importance of timing, and positioning … all useful information for preparation for doing announcement at home.
- **Observed practice** focuses on the physical, relational and reflective responses within and outside the group work sessions. Sarah noted that she had tried many other interventions but found the NVR approach helpful as she was participating with other parents who were enduring similar challenges. In addition, the opportunities of learning from feedback, performing and hearing the views of other parents brought forth an intervention that was specific, situated and contextually useful.

 

## Practice ideas to facilitate coaching

Below are some ideas that can help facilitate the framework for safeguarding practice with parents:

- Encourage parents to develop the confidence to show and tell how they are applying and relating NVR ideas to practice.
- Facilitators should model the performance of the ideas. An example would be the performance of escalation and de-escalation within their immediate context.
- Facilitators should create a context where the tools are continually evaluated, monitored and reviewed. Anecdotal experience from facilitating NVR parenting groups suggest that parents value practising the tools within their context and giving feedback on how they experience acting into the doing of the ideas – focusing on what works, what they might do differently and why.
- Encourage the idea of respect for each participant's contribution. There is no set way of performing NVR principles: this will be unique and specific to each parent and their situated context.
- Create an expectation of change, which could include the motivation to try the NVR tools and seeing what happens, as one example.
- Nurture the idea of connection and the rebuilding of relationships and the importance of being with the other rather than having power over the other.
- Sustaining progress, create opportunities for an on-going group which parents can access long after they have completed the course.

## Conclusion

As an approach, NVR is still in its infancy in the UK and has yet to be endorsed by the National Institute for Health and Care Excellence (NICE), so it does not carry the evidence-based practice seal of approval. However, Munro *et al* (2016) draw attention to the need to re-consider our relationship with evidence-based ideas as well as other sources of information, as they argue that evidence-based ideas are often not complete or sufficient to deal with the complexity of safeguarding and the uniqueness of each family's situated context. This is one of the elements that makes the NVR approach particularly valuable. NVR has the flexibility to work alongside the uniqueness of the family's situation and can be used both within an individual and a group context.

However, Preston-Shoot (2007) observes that group work can be arduous, making it an unattractive form of intervention, and adds that claims for effectiveness are not that substantial in terms of evidence-based practice. He stresses the importance of locating the evidence for group work's relevance and value and sees this as imperative.

Sarah's account (p69) is not unique and many more are documented in the parents' booklet, *Non-Violent Resistance* (Oxleas NHS Foundation Trust, 2013). In addition, there is a steady growth of research in Europe (Van Holen *et al*, 2015) that shows the effectiveness of NVR. But this is not yet the case in the UK where the process and structure of undertaking research tends to favour research design that is supported by positive methodologies, as indicated by Munro *et al* (2016), who raise concerns that, 'People turn to empirical research because they see the rigor of scientific methods as contributing more reliable knowledge for welfare services' (p3).

Munro *et al* (2016) join many other scholars (Bateson, 2016; Todes, 2007; Feyerabend, 1987) who argue that scientific research, situated at the top end of the hierarchy of evidence-based practice, is not the only method that can produce valuable knowledge. Within the domain of evidence-based practice, the issue of expert knowledge is valued over local knowledge, which goes against the emerging NVR discourse which is situated within a systemic, social constructionist and postmodernist frame. These discourses share a commonality that banishes the idea of expert knowledge, where the expert is usually a clinical/ professional who has competency and mastery of skills. Within the NVR approach, everyone is deemed to have expertise in their own situation, and moreover, the idea is that multiple knowledge is privileged over knowledge emerging from the single voice of the clinician. That said, within a social care context, for example, NVR acknowledges the importance of safeguarding and thus creates space for numerous conversations to be had that are visible and tangible (Dalzell & Sawyer, 2016) rather than abstract. In this way they can be discussed, which invites the process of reflexivity (Burnham, 2005; Burnham & Neden, 2007); not as a position where one is validating what one already knows but going beyond 'comfortable reflection' to 'reflection of discomfort'.

I want to end by proposing that NVR provides a way forward by coaching parents to safeguard their children. The practice skill set offers relational rules which affirm practice but also encourage and invite parents to engage in a practical discourse which is visible, present, observable and intuitive. NVR coaching encourages parents to use the skills developed within their own natural environment so they can be better integrated and adapted to fit their specific purpose. Parents are encouraged to become acquainted with their social world through participation, engagement and by developing a shared understanding with others.

The coaching style of the NVR approach makes the practice visible within the individual context, but in addition, the performance of the activities within a group of other parents with similar issues creates a sense of membership (Wenger, 2008), a collective core which in turn creates a sense of community, belonging and motivation. The co-joint collaborative partnership between practitioners and graduate parents is a move towards a collaborative and appreciative form of practice. This creates a space for shared knowledge, both from clinicians and graduate parents, to co-exist and flourish from the mingling of multiple experiences. The lived experiences of graduate parents and the learned experiences of the group facilitators creates a pool of knowledge acquired through the complex and creative exchanges in the group process. This offers a contribution that focuses on ways of doing and telling that connect with the everyday life of all the participants. Supporting parents to be wise parents was one of the ideas echoed by Munro (2011). We argue that the NVR approach can provide a way for parents to become better able to safeguard their children.

## References

Bateson N (2016) *Small Arcs of Larger Circles: Framing through.* Axminster, England: Triarchy Press.

Burnham JB (2005) Relational reflexivity: a tool for socially constructing therapeutic relationships. In: C Flaskas, B Mason & A Perlesz (Eds.) *The Space Between: Experience, context, and process in the therapeutic relationship* (p1-17). London: Karnac.

Burnham JB & Neden J (2007) Using relational reflexivity as a resource in teaching family therapy. *Journal of Family Therapy* **29** (4) p359–363.

Condry R & Miles C (2012) Adolescent to parent violence and youth justice in England and Wales. *Social Policy and Society* **11** p241–250

Condry R & Miles C (2013) Adolescent to parent violence: framing and mapping a hidden problem. *British Society of Criminology and Criminal Justice* **14** (3) p257–275.

Coogan D (2012) Marking the boundaries – when troublesome becomes abuse and children cross a line in family violence. *Journal of the Family Therapy Association of Ireland*. p74-87.

Dalzell R & Sawyer E (2016) *Putting Analysis into Child and Family Assessment*. London: Jessica Kingsley Publishers.

Day EM & Heismann E (2010) *Non-Violent Resistance Programme: For all those working with parents and carers of children and adolescents with violent behaviours*. Brighton & Hove: Pavilion Publishing & Media Ltd.

Dewey J (1934) *Art as Experience* (1958, 6th ed.). New York: Capricorn.

Etherington K (2007) Ethical Research in Reflexive relationship. *Journal of Qualitative Inquiry* **13** (5) pp599–616.

Gilad Z (2017) Presentation given on 'Parent Patrol'. NVR Conference, London 2017.

Feyerabend P (1987) *Farewell to Reason.* New York: Verso.

Firmin C (2017) Contextualizing case reviews: a methodology for developing systemic safeguarding practices. *Child and Family Social Work*. DOI:10.1111/cfa.12382.

Ford R (2015) Parents call in police to control their children. *The Times* **10 March**. Available at: https://www.thetimes.co.uk/article/parents-call-in-police-to-control-their-children-xvqhftwpbvg (accessed September 2018).

Forrester D, Westlake D, McCannn A, Thurham A, Shefer G, Glynn G & Killian M (2013) *Reclaiming Social Work? An evaluation of systemic units as an approach to delivering children's services.*

Gallwey WT (1986) *The Inner Game of Tennis: The ultimate guide to the mental side of peak performance*. United Kingdom: Pans Book

Gergen KJ (2009) *Relational Being: Beyond self and community*. Oxford & New York. University Press.

Goodman S & Trowler I (2012) *Social Work Reclaimed: Innovative frameworks for child and family social work practice.* London: Jessica Kingsley Publishers.

Higashia N (2017) *Fall Down 7 Times get up 8: A young man's voice from the silence of Autism*. London Hodder & Stoughton Ltd.

Levinas E (2006) *Humanism of the Other.* Urbana & Chicago. University of Illinois Press.

Laming H (2003) *The Victoria Climbié Inquiry: Report of an inquiry by Lord Laming*. London: The Stationery Office.

Merleau-Ponty M (1983) *The Structure of Behaviour.* Alden L Fisher, Pittsburgh: Duquesne University Press.

Munro E, Cartwright N, Hardie J & Montuschi E (2016) *Improving Child Safety: Deliberation, judgement and empirical research*. CHESS. Durham University.

Munro E (2011) *The Munro Review of Child Protection: Final Report. A child-centred system* [online]. London: Department for Education.

Munro E, Taylor JS & Bradbury-Jones C (2013) Understanding the causal pathways to child maltreatment: implications for health and social care policy and practice. *Child Abuse Review* **23** (1) p61–74.

Newman M, Fagan C & Webb R (2014) Innovations in practice: the efficacy of nonviolent resistance groups in treating aggressive and controlling children and young people: a preliminary analysis of pilot NVR groups in Kent. *Child and Adolescent Mental Health* **19** (2) p138–141.

NSPCC (2014) *On the Edge: Childline spotlight* [online]. Available at: www.nspcc.org.uk/services-and-resources/research-and-resources/on-the-edge-ChildLine-spotlight/ (accessed September 2018).

Omer H (2004) *Non-Violent Resistance: A new approach to violent and self- destructive children*. Cambridge: Cambridge University Press.

Omer H (2011) *The New Authority: Family, school and community*. Cambridge: Cambridge University Press.

Oxleas NHS Foundation Trust (2013) *Non-Violent Resistance. NVR – Rebuilding Family Relationships. Testimonies from parents, family members and supporters. How NVR has helped change life in my family.* Oxleas NHS Foundation Trust.

Pona I, Royston S, Bracey C & Gibbs A (2015) Seriously Awkward: How vulnerable 16-17 year olds are falling through the cracks [online]. London: The Children's Society. Available at: https://www.childrenssociety.org.uk/sites/default/files/seriously_awkward_youth-at-risk_full_online-final-new.pdf (accessed September 2018).

Pillow W (2003) Confession, catharsis, or cure? Rethinking the uses of reflexivity as methodological power in qualitative research. *International Journal of Qualitative Studies in Education* **16** (2) p175–196.

Preston-Shoot M (2007) *Effective Groupwork Work* (2nd ed). London and New York: Palgrave Macmillan.

 

Preston-Shoot M (2017) What is really wrong with serious case reviews? *Child Abuse Review.* Wiley Online Library. DOI: 10.1002/car.2487.

Schatzki T, Cetina KK & Savigny von E (2001) *The Practice Turn in Contemporary Theory*. London and New York: Routledge.

Searle J (1969) *Speech Acts: An essay in the philosophy of language.* Cambridge: Cambridge University Press.

Shotter J (2016) *Speaking, Actually: Towards a new 'fluid common-sense understanding of relational becomings*. Farnhill: Everything is Connected Press.

Starhawk (1987) *Truth or Dare: Encounters with power, authority, and mystery.* San Francisco: Harper.

Todes l (2007) *Embodied Enquiry: Phenomenological touchstones for research, psychotherapy, and spirituality*. Basingstoke: Palgrave Macmillan.

Van Holen F, Vanderfaeillie J & Omer H (2015) Adaptation and evaluation of a nonviolent resistance intervention for foster parents: A progress report. *Journal of Marital and Family Therapy* doi:10.1111/jmft.12125.

Weinblatt U & Omer H (2008) Non-violent resistance: a treatment for parents for children with acute behaviour problems. *Journal of Marital and Family Therapy* **34** p75–92.

Wenger E (2008) *Communities of Practice: Learning, meaning and identity (Learning in Doing: Social, Cognitive and Computational Perspectives).* USA: Cambridge University Press.

Wittgenstein L (1953) *Philosophical Investigations*, trans. G.E.M. Anscombe, Oxford: Blackwell.

Wood A (2016) *Wood Report: Review of the role and functions of local safeguarding children boards.* The Stationery Office: London.

# Chapter 6: Using NVR in adult mental health services

By Linda Cakebread

## Introduction

As a graduate NVR parent facilitator, I have found it useful to teach NVR techniques to some parents and carers of users of adult mental health services where I now work. Many mental health problems affecting children, such as autism spectrum disorder (ASD), attention deficit hyperactivity disorder (ADHD), obsessive compulsive disorder (OCD), phobias, anxiety and depression, continue into adulthood, and the problems facing the parents of these children do not stop simply because their child reaches adulthood.

As well as unacceptable behaviours, there is also a tendency for the adult child to remain overly dependent on parents, which can often lead to unreasonable demands on them. The parents, meanwhile, may believe that their adult child is unable to care for themselves or to function without their help. Such 'giving in' by the parents often means that the adult child continues to remain dysfunctional and fails to learn to care for themselves (Lebowitz *et al*, 2012), and the parents are left coping with the same problems they had when their 'children' were children.

While working with some of these parents, as well as carers of other adult family members who have become overly dependent on them due to mental ill health, I noticed the similarities between them and the parents I see when co-facilitating NVR groups within child and adolescent mental health services (CAMHS). This led me to believe that NVR techniques could be useful to these parents and carers of adults as well.

In this chapter I will be describing a case I have worked on and explaining how it has helped both the parent and the adult child they care for. (I will not be using the client or parent's real names in order to protect their anonymity.) I will also describe how I adapt the NVR programme in order to use the techniques with adult children rather than children.

## How NVR helped me

I was introduced to NVR through CAMHS in 2011 due to problems in my family, and I found the course so useful that I regularly attended the parent support group run by other graduate parents and then signed up as a volunteer graduate parent co-facilitator. I also started volunteering in other areas of my local NHS health trust and participated in training with them as a Lived Experience Practitioner (LXP). I now work part time in a paid role as an LXP in adult mental health.

I base a lot of my NVR work on my own experience as a parent. When she was young, my daughter struggled with anxiety and depression for several years and was self-harming and took several overdoses. She did not make friends easily, but aged 14 she began to spend time with a crowd at the local shopping centre who took advantage of her vulnerability. She thought they were her friends, but she had to 'buy' their friendship by selling her possessions and shoplifting to provide them with money and stolen goods. They encouraged her to start smoking cigarettes which then progressed to smoking cannabis.

By this point our relationship was strained, and since I had never been able to understand her self-harm, we didn't really talk about what was going on. I was also afraid to tackle her about her behaviour for fear that any arguments would lead her to self-harm. We had never really had much success with her engaging with CAMHS so when her care co-ordinator suggested I try the NVR group I thought it was worth a try.

I attended the course and noticed changes quite early on. As my relationship with my daughter improved through de-escalation and reconciliation gestures, she felt I was listening to her more and therefore opened up to me more. As the whole situation at home began to improve, my confidence in myself and my ability as a parent grew (helped by the fact that the self-announcement had helped me to let go of the guilt I felt and to stop blaming myself for everything) and we moved on from the past. Although she still has problems with anxiety and depression, she no longer self-harms and our relationship is much better.

## How I use NVR in my work today

The service users under the team I work in usually have diagnoses such as schizophrenia or bipolar disorders, or may not yet have a definitive diagnosis. These types of illness can result in people becoming less able to look after themselves and more reliant on their family or friends to care for them. Sometimes however, even when the illness is better controlled and the symptoms less severe, the service user can be left feeling anxious and vulnerable and still feeling they need to rely on the care of others. Their parents/carers, because of their compassion for the person and their desire to help, therefore continue to provide their support, which they deem to be necessary. However this does not allow the person to attempt things for themselves, or free themselves from depending on others, which they may well succeed in given the opportunity (Lebowitz, 2016).

When I began working in adult mental health as an LXP, I wasn't sure how I could use NVR in my work as it was all based around families and children. However, I noticed that despite my own family being grown up, I was still using NVR with them. It was at this time that I was asked to work with a few parents/carers of my colleagues' adult clients because they were struggling to cope and my colleagues knew I was a carer myself. I began working with these carers on a one-to-one basis and noticed the similarities between them and the parents I saw at CAMHS groups. They had the same difficulties such as the demands being made on them, i.e. to do things like cooking and cleaning, giving lifts or dealing with paperwork and making phone calls. Like teenagers, these clients were often isolating themselves in their rooms and neglecting their social lives, for example, rather than going out with friends.

I had already begun teaching some NVR tools to the parents/carers I saw when I begun researching the use of NVR with adults who remain dependent on their parents. I then decided to structure the work I do individually with them, a little more like the group course is delivered.

The first thing I do with parents/carers is to explain that the work is targeted at them and that the person they care for does not have to engage with services or any therapy (often a problem, as many dependent adults either do not realise there is a problem or feel that no therapy will work and so refuse to accept help from professionals).

I also explain that although the work is directed at them, they are not being blamed, shamed or judged for the way they have handled things until this point. This is a very important message, as many such parents will blame themselves – it's easy to get 'stuck' with feelings of guilt for past mistakes, which leaves a person unable to move on and do anything about their current situation. I explain that they are simply being taught different ways to deal with the challenging or demanding person they care for. I always emphasise that they are not being accused of doing things the 'wrong' way, but simply that if the way they are doing things is not working, it's worth trying something new.

## Adult Entitled Dependence

In 2009, Haim Omer used the term 'Adult Entitled Dependence' (AED) to describe the emotional dependence of adult offspring on their parents, leading to dysfunction and distress. AED is defined as a 'chronic, family systemic condition involving a dysfunctional adult offspring and at least one parent who accommodates to the patterns of dependence by providing age-inappropriate services' (Tel-Aviv Center for NVR Psychology, 2018). Lebowitz *et al* (2012) describe their work with the parents of 27 adult-dependent children (using the term AED) and how NVR training can help those parents to break out of the situation they are in. They describe how the child's escalating demands lead to the parents giving in, which leads in turn to both parents and child believing that the child cannot cope on their own and therefore the parents must continue to accommodate their child's 'needs'. After parents completed the programme, many of the adult children went on to move into independent accommodation and gain employment.

Norman *et al* (2015) examined studies in childhood anxiety and found that many of the subjects did not engage with or respond to treatment. They describe how parental accommodation of the child's perceived needs contributes to the child's ongoing anxiety. The Supportive Parenting for Anxious Childhood Emotions (SPACE) program addressed this issue, targeting children's anxiety without requiring the child to participate. SPACE works with the parents to reduce parental accommodation and the problems it causes. Trials of SPACE have been completed for youths with OCD (Lebowitz, 2013) and paediatric anxiety disorders (Lebowitz *et al*, 2014). They then went on to use a modified form of NVR and found it reduced parental accommodation, and therefore some of the symptoms of anxious and overly dependent young adults. These young adults increased their independent functioning and the parents were able to involve more support for themselves and the adult dependant.

## Working with Anne

One specific carer I worked with was a mother who I will refer to as Anne, whose son had suffered a psychotic episode a couple of years previously and been in hospital for several months. Before this time he had been working and was quite independent. On his return from hospital he remained quite depressed and became anxious about several things. When I saw Anne she was quite worn down by the constant care she had to provide for her son and by worrying about him. He made no attempts to improve his situation himself, even refusing any therapy, in the belief that nothing would work. Anne and her husband had separated but both still lived in the family home, unwilling to sell the house for fear of what would happen to their son.

## De-escalation

The first technique I usually introduce is de-escalation, but when I mentioned this to Anne she explained that her son did not argue and was not aggressive. However, he did have a tendency to 'grab' her every time he saw her and dominate her time by going over his problems again and again with her. Although Anne felt that she had a good relationship with her son, on reflection she realised that these conversations were not healthy for either of them. So I used this as the point to 'de-escalate' by encouraging her to try not to get drawn into them, telling her son that she would talk to him later (when he was calmer and less emotional). Although he still continued to try to talk to her in this way, she found she was able to limit these types of conversations so they happened less frequently.

## Reconciliation gestures

I usually also introduce reconciliation gestures at this point in order to repair any damage in the relationship between them. As in NVR with children, a large part of the process is about re-connecting parents/carers with the person they care for and rebuilding their relationship. This can be achieved partly by de-escalating highly emotional situations and partly by offering reconciliation gestures unrelated to behaviour, to let the person know that they are still loved and cared about even though their carer is treating them differently.

## Connnecting and resisting comments

Both of these tools are usually accompanied with a newer NVR concept used in some CAMHS groups – see Chapter 18. Once a situation has been de-escalated, these conversations are a good tool to 'strike while the iron is cold' and to begin to tackle problems without re-escalating the situation.

## Parental presence and siblings

The next technique usually taught in CAMHS groups is parental presence. In this instance the parental presence in the son was more that of his mother being there to take care of him and be his emotional sounding board rather than not being there. So I felt this was more about Anne getting her own personal presence back and making an independent life for herself, hoping that her example may be observed and learned by her son.

At this time we also usually introduce the subject of siblings. This applies less often to parents and carers of adults, as quite often any siblings are already living independently and may not be aware that their parent is using NVR. However, where siblings do live in the home it is useful to explain NVR to some degree, as quite often they see their sibling's behaviour negatively and feel that the parent's use of de-escalation is simply 'giving in'. They therefore need to be made aware of the techniques being used, and it is also possible that they can perhaps apply them themselves, or simply support the parent/carers in what they are doing. In Anne's case there was another son who had recently left home, so I encouraged Anne to explain some of the techniques she was using with him so that he would understand and be more supportive.

## The baskets technique

'The baskets' technique of prioritising is always useful, and I find I use it in a lot of different areas of my life – whenever you have a lot to deal with and you don't know where to start, write down all of the problems separately and put them into baskets. Using this technique, a parent or carer can prioritise the issues in their relationship with their child and can pinpoint the biggest/or most damaging behaviour to concentrate on first. Following this technique, just one or two behaviours are placed into the smallest basket – the most significant issues to be focused on first. In the middle basket are the behaviours that can perhaps be negotiated on, while the largest basket contains all the less serious behaviours that will not be responded to at present. Once the problems in the small basket have improved, there may be opportunity to move items up from the medium basket to replace them.

Once the smaller, less impactful behaviours have been put in the large basket, it is much easier to concentrate on the one or two most important aspects of the situation. In the same way as the concept is explained to parents of children using NVR, this is usually based on the parents/carer's values. The top priority is often based on safety. Another high priority with parents/carers of adults is often helping the adult to become more independent. The use of a fourth basket (the rainbow basket) to list all the good things about the adult and things that make the parent/carer love them, can help to remind them why they are trying to help their dependent adult. In this case, as with most parents, Anne was trying to make everything perfect for her son, which would be impossible. Instead, I encouraged her to prioritise the things that were the most important – for Anne, that was her son's constant need to go over and over the past with her and his reluctance to leave the house at all. This narrowed things down a bit for her so she was not trying to deal with too much at the same time.

## Self-care and supporters

Next comes a very important step, particularly for the parents and carers of dependent adults – self-care and supporters. Parents/carers of adults are usually a little bit older than parents of children, and most would not have expected to be looking after someone else at this stage, whether that be an adult 'child' or a sibling or partner. This can make it harder to cope with. Self-care is also important as it can increase the mental and emotional resilience of the parent/carer, giving them greater capacity for continuing with the NVR techniques and persevering to resolve the issues in their relationships.

Self-care is therefore extremely important, and one important aspect of self-care is the use of supporters. In my work, I not only help parents/carers to identify who their supporters are but also to determine what type of supporters they are and how they can be 'used'. Some supporters are able to offer a sympathetic ear while others can offer more practical help and support. It may also be useful to have a supporter learn the principles of NVR, too, so that they can help to support the parent/carer when implementing them.

Anne felt she had a number of supporters. Firstly there was the boy's father, her ex-husband – however until then they had both been dealing with their son in different ways. I therefore got her to go through some of the NVR techniques with him and get him on board so they were both 'on the same page'. This helped enormously and Anne no longer feels so alone in trying to deal with their son. She also had friends with whom she spent quite a bit of time outside the home, a practice I encouraged her to continue. She felt, however, that although these friends were very supportive they did not really understand what it was like to live with an adult dependant, so she still felt quite alone at times. This is where doing the NVR course as part of a group would really be useful, so that she could meet other parents/carers in similar situations.

## Self-announcement and announcement

Writing a self-announcement can also be important to help parents/carers identify anything that may be holding them back. As mentioned, there may often be feelings of guilt and self-blame about how they have dealt with things in the past or not coped very well (Weinblatt, 2013). Parents in particular often blame themselves for bringing their children up in a certain way or in a certain environment. Anne seemed to feel that she was to blame for doing too much for her son when he became ill and not helping him to regain his independence earlier. I explained to her, in the way it was explained to me, that anything we have done in the past we did because we thought we were doing the right thing at the time. We didn't do it purposely to harm or damage our children in any way and therefore we should not blame ourselves for the way things have turned out. Furthermore, holding on to guilt and ruminating over what we should have done differently simply holds us back and stops us from moving on. Once Anne had written a self-announcement she realised she could leave the past where it belonged, in the past, and concentrate on changing the present and the future.

Then comes the announcement to the person concerned. I encouraged Anne to write an announcement stating that she would no longer be sitting in his room for hours listening to him ruminating over the past. She pointed out that this behaviour was harmful to him and therefore she was going to do this for his own good because she loves him and cares about him. This also ties in with active resistance. Some of the problems with adults are the same as with children, or teenagers in particular, where they expect everything to be done for them, not because they expect it as their right but because they feel unable to do things for themselves. I therefore encouraged Anne to resist her son's requests for hours of her time by a) talking with him only 'by appointment' at specific times, b) limiting the length of time for these talks and c) encouraging her son to come down to the living room to talk rather than stay shut away in his bedroom.

## The sit-in

The sit-in that is usually part of the NVR course is not always necessary if the other tools outlined in this chapter are working. But if things have not improved it may be necessary to get the parent/carer to sit with the person and remind them of the announcement and the behaviour in question and ask that they try to come up with a solution. In this case, Anne used the sit-in, which led to her son beginning to think more for himself about what he could do about his own situation instead of relying on her to provide all the answers. Most adults are, in fact, more likely to co-operate and try to make changes if they are involved in the decisions about how to implement them in the first place.

# Summary

All these techniques together have had a positive overall impact on the family. Anne and her husband, although no longer together, are both dealing with their son in the same way and therefore being more supportive of each other, offering a more solid foundation for their son to build his future on. Anne is feeling much better about her own life and was able to move on, having realised that her son could manage without her always being there. And her son has begun to do more for himself and ruminate on the past much less.

As a graduate parent co-facilitator, I've realised how important graduate parents are to the NVR programme. Professional NVR facilitators who have worked both with and without graduate parents often comment on how they achieve much better results with new parents when graduate parents are co-facilitating. New parents 'buy in' to the whole concept of NVR a lot more quickly and easily because they have the graduate parents' testimonies on how NVR has worked for them.

Graduate parents who have found NVR useful in their own lives and want to come back as volunteer co-facilitators are usually very passionate about NVR, and that passion clearly shows when they talk about their experiences of using the techniques. They often tell new parents how difficult their lives were before NVR and how their situation has since been greatly improved.

As discussed, parents often come to NVR with feelings of guilt, perhaps feeling they have been 'bad' parents or that they have behaved the wrong way or allowed things to happen in their and/or their children's lives. Graduate parents can explain to parents who feel this way in a manner that perhaps professionals who have not actually used NVR techniques in their own personal lives cannot; how there are no judgements being made about them as parents; that there can be difficulties with children no matter what parents have done or whether they've been 'good' or 'bad'.

NVR is not a magic cure or the answer to all their problems, but it can realistically improve at least some of the difficulties they experience and can make them feel better about themselves and how they are handling things, making them stronger and better able to cope.

These are concepts which are difficult to explain without being able to give real-life examples demonstrating exactly how it works. Certainly, in my work I use my own experience to illustrate these points, however, this experience is limited to my particular situation. The benefit of working within groups is that we would have several graduate parents whose situations were different, and therefore the range of experience covered would be wider and it would be more likely that a 'story' will resonate with each of the parents. When I set up an NVR course for parents/carers of adults I will bring in some of the graduate parent volunteers from CAMHS as there are a number whose children are now adults and who, like me, still use NVR with them.

Another advantage of the CAMHS groups is that the parents also have monthly support groups which they run themselves. There are no professionals at these meetings so parents can discuss their problems freely, although there is usually a professional on hand if needed and the facilitators have a debrief after the group to discuss any safeguarding issues or any worries that parents might have. This is something that could also be set up by parents/carers of adults after they have graduated from an NVR course, to give them continued support.

From working with parents/carers on a one-to-one basis I have found that they often feel very alone. Even though they may have support from friends and family, those supporters do not really understand what it is like to live with an adult with these issues and behaviours. This is where the NVR course for groups of parents/carers would be useful because, as well as teaching the valuable NVR techniques, it also puts parents/carers in touch with each other and means they see others going through the same problems, reducing that sense of isolation. This alone helps parents/carers to cope better and feel stronger, which means they are much more capable of using NVR techniques successfully.

## Looking forward

My next steps will be to present my ideas and the concepts of NVR and the NVR course to the team in which I work. My NVR lead from CAMHS has agreed to help me with this presentation, which I believe will add more weight to it and get people interested in the ideas of NVR who prefer to listen to professionals rather than parent experts by experience. Along with some personal testimonies and some data around how NVR helps and produces results, I hope to get several team members on board with the project.

After identifying those team members who will work on the project, they will need training. There are several options for this but one of the first steps will be to get them to shadow the professionals in CAMHS as they deliver an NVR course, so they can learn how to deliver the program themselves. Once trained, we can then start looking at the practicalities i.e. venues, times, numbers, target groups etc. Then we will write up some referral specifications and distribute to the team, and perhaps give another presentation for care co-ordinators to learn a bit more about the course so they can discuss it with their client's parents/carers. After making all the arrangements and deciding on our participants, invitations will be sent getting them along to an introductory session where we would sign up those who are interested. We would have to do pre- and after-course assessments to measure outcomes to show that the course is viable and worth continuing.

Ideally, I would continue to follow the progress of the participants and their cared-for adults to research how well the course is working and if the intervention has a long-term impact on the clients themselves. As we have discovered with our work in schools, it helps if teachers and schools use (or are at least aware of) NVR alongside the parents. It may therefore be a good idea to bring NVR into adult mental health services more widely, i.e. staff on wards or in the home treatment and community teams. Some of the techniques could be useful, particularly on the inpatient wards, but it would be helpful for more staff to know about the techniques in order to support parents and carers.

 

# References

Lebowitz ER, Dolberger D, Nortov E & Omer H (2012) Parent training in nonviolent resistance for adult entitled dependence. *Family Process* **51**(1) 90–106.

Lebowitz ER (2013) Parent-based treatment for childhood and adolescent OCD. *Journal of Obsessive-Compulsive and Related Disorders* **2** (4) 425–431.

Lebowitz ER, Omer H, Hermes H & Scahill L (2014) Parent training for childhood anxiety disorders: The SPACE program. *Cognitive and Behavioral Practice* **21** (4) 456–469.

Lebowitz ER (2016) "Failure to Launch": Shaping intervention for highly dependent adult children. *Journal of the American Academy of Child and Adolescent Psychiatry* **55**(2) 89–90

Norman K, Silverman WK & Lebowitz ER (2015) Family accommodation of child and adolescent anxiety: mechanisms, assessment and treatment. *Journal of Child and Adolescent Psychiatric Nursing* **28** (3) 131–140.

Tel-Aviv Center for NVR Psychology (2018) *Adult Entitled Dependence: Failure to Emerge: Extreme social withdrawal, dependence and emerging adulthood* [online]. Available at: http://nvrpsy.com/adult-entitled-dependence/what-is-aed/ (accessed September 2018).

Weinblatt U (2013) Regulating shame in intense parent-child conflict through the use of public opinion in NVR therapy. *Familiendynamik* **38** (1) 62–71.

# Chapter 7: More than just a good idea? From practice to scientific underpinning

**Frank Van Holen and Johan Vanderfaeillie**

## Introduction

Non-violent resistance (NVR) and New Authority (NA) have found their way into an increasing number of care settings, and the areas and target groups to which they can be applied continue to broaden. This chapter takes a critical look at both NVR and NA. First, we argue why NVR and NA are intervention programmes (referred to here as 'interventions'). Next we discuss how NVR and NA relate to each other[1]. We make a distinction between what is support and what is an *intervention*. We then make an analysis of these two approaches based on five basic questions (Vanderfaeillie & Van Holen, 2010):

1. Who uses them?
2. What are the goals?
3. Who administers them?
4. What do they consist of?
5. What do they yield?

We end with a conclusion and a presentation of a future research agenda.

1 In some communities, the concept of the NA has not been adopted. Important aspects from NA are integrated into NVR. In these communities, compared to international literature, NVR is considered a broader framework which embraces ideas of vigilant care and makes the approach applicable to a wide range of authority figures, preventive as well as curative. In this chapter, however, we clarify the relationship between NVR and NA in order to introduce readers to the concepts which they will confront in the literature.

## NVR and NA as therapeutic interventions

We begin by describing what an intervention is. At the most basic level, an intervention consists of adapting or altering the behaviours of care providers (e.g. consulting with parents as to which behaviour/s will no longer be acceptable). At a higher level, an intervention is a specific technique (e.g. preparing, writing and reading the announcement together are the constituent parts of the technique 'the announcement'). A collection of techniques, at a still higher level, form the methodology of the intervention (e.g. actions of resistance to problem behaviour combined with relationship gestures, emotion regulation and seeking support). The methodology forms the total package of the intervention, together with any implementation requirements such as the length of treatment, its frequency and intensity (Van Yperen *et al*, 2008).

It is assumed that NVR and NA are interventions and the five basic questions set out in the introduction are used to explore this. Through careful reading of numerous publications by Omer, colleagues and other researchers (e.g. Omer, 2004; 2011; Omer & Lebowitz, 2016; Omer *et al*, 2008), we conclude that NVR is an intervention in the sense that we have described. With the wide use of the terms 'application' (Omer, 2004, pIX) and 'treatment method' (Lavi-Levavi *et al*, 2013, p79; Omer & Lebowitz, 2016, p698) in the literature, and in particular by providing a manual for parents (Omer, 2004), it is clear that Omer and many others in the field consider NVR to be an intervention. Moreover, in other publications, NVR is described as a 'parent-training programme' (Omer *et al*, 2008, p450), an 'NVR-training' (Lavi-Levavi *et al*, 2013, p92), and a 'transdiagnostic treatment' (Omer & Lebowitz, 2016, p698).

However, some ambiguity is created when trying to define a practical, detailed and consistent *theory* (Omer, 2004, pIX), a translation and application of the *doctrine* of NVR against violent and self-destructive children and adolescents (Omer, 2004, pIX; Omer & Lebowitz, 2016, p688), an *attitude* that contains a number of principles (Omer, 2001, p65) and a *philosophy* (Lavi-Levavi *et al*, 2013, p80) behind the approach.

With NA (Omer, 2011), a broader framework was created. It can be seen as an extension of NVR in four key ways:

1. The initial focus primarily on parents is extended to encompass all parenting and authority figures including teachers, residential group workers, youth police etc.
2. The word 'resistance' in NVR mainly concerns a *reaction* to unacceptable behaviours. With NA, a preventive element is added (Shachar-Lavi, 2011).

 

3. NVR addresses serious problem behaviour that renders parents helpless and gives them the feeling that they have to adapt to and accept these behaviours. With NA, situations are included in which the vigilance of parenting figures is relevant, with issues such as lying, bad company, truancy, smoking, alcohol and drugs, unsafe sex, diabetes, computer abuse, unsafe driving, etc. (Omer & Lebowitz, 2016).
4. NVR is embedded in a more general pedagogical model (e.g. Bom & Wiebenga, 2017; Omer *et al*, 2017). The core of NA is vigilant care (Amiel, 2011; Omer, 2011), a dynamic and fluctuating process that provides parents with guidelines for how to act across a range of escalating parenting problems (Omer, 2011). Vigilant care comprises three levels: having an open dialogue with the child, asking them focused questions and taking unilateral actions (Omer, 2011).

In relation to this fourth point, the first level of providing vigilant care involves parenting behaviours such as non-intrusive and loving attention. With NA, parents are given the tools to supervise their children in an age-appropriate way, to have open, honest and spontaneous conversations with their children, and to discuss difficult topics. Simultaneously, rules and expectations are clearly formulated and discussed with their children (Omer *et al*, 2017). This attitude is similar to authoritative parenting as described by Baumrind (1971), and by Maccoby and Martin (1983) (see Omer *et al*, 2017). In short, by overlapping the first level of vigilant care with authoritative parenting, NVR and NA are embedded in a positive and effective parenting style.

The second level of vigilant care involves parents learning and watching out for warning signals that require increased vigilance. Parental figures are supported and instructed in focused supervision.

At the third level of vigilant care, parental figures are supported to undertake unilateral actions when serious problems arise.

Vigilant care therefore comes down to supporting parents to provide authoritative parenting, in which, depending on warning signals and risks, they shift between these three levels (Omer *et al*, 2017). Omer *et al* (2013, p197) state: *'The greater the parents' ability to shift between the three levels of vigilant care, the more effective is his or her authority'*.

NA can also be called an intervention. At the first level, it concerns the stimulation of authoritative parenthood, and is very much in line with forms of parenting support and early parenting education to help parents raise their children in an authoritative way. This parenting style results in socially competent children and young people who demonstrate few problem behaviours (Lamborn *et al*, 1991).

The second and third levels are only addressed in case of warning signals (second level), or serious problems (third level). With the second level, a preventive component is added with methodology manuals, depending on the problem and risk conditions (Omer *et al*, 2016). Although the concrete techniques differ, these programmes are based on experiences gained with NVR-interventions: *'These programmes drew from previous experience on how to help parents cope with violent and self-destructive behaviours through nonviolent resistance, which involves a combination of decided parental presence, prevention of escalation, and minimisation of control messages'* (Omer *et al*, 2017, p298). However, it is not always clear in the literature which programmes are situated at the second preventive level or at the third curative level. Moreover, the terms NVR, NA and vigilant care are often used in an undifferentiated and interchangeable way.

## How do NVR and NA relate to each other?

In the previous section we indicated that NA can be seen as a broader framework in which NVR has a place. We called the first level, the open dialogue, a form of upbringing *support*. The second and third levels were named *intervention* forms that use techniques originally developed for the NVR-intervention. We will now go deeper into the connections between NVR and NA in relation to the continuum of parenting problems (ordinary upbringing – upbringing tension – problematic upbringing situation).

The first level of vigilant care aims to encourage parents to acquire knowledge about their children through spontaneous communication. It encourages parents to invest time in their children, to create a faithful atmosphere and to show interest in their children in a positive way. This ensures that parents and children develop a positive and trusting relationship. Attention, presence and protection by the parent are encouraged (Omer, 2011). Activities that aim to disseminate such advice to parents can be called parenting *support*. Parenting support is indeed a collective term for all activities aimed at optimising and improving parenting skills, with the most important aim being to prevent more serious (parenting) problems from developing. Parents are encouraged in their self-dependence and in increasing their skills as parenting figures (Burggraaff-Huiskes, 2007).

This raises a question about the nature of the upbringing that NA is aiming at. In several places it becomes clear that Omer opts for authoritative upbringing (Omer *et al*, 2013; Omer *et al*, 2017) characterised by high levels of warmth and responsiveness on the one hand, and expectations and supervision (demandingness) on the other hand. 'Parental responsiveness' refers to the amount of support and affection between parents and child. Responsiveness also includes a second aspect – that parents are able to alleviate discomfort and tensions in the child (Baumrind, 2013; Janssens, 1986; Maccoby & Martin, 1983).

Concerning *demandingness*, authoritative parenting figures have clear expectations and they dare to make demands. They structure the behaviour of their child with clear rules. They explain why these rules are important. In the event of a violation, an adequate response is given. All this is done through open communication. Parents take into account the opinion of their child, but also clearly state their own (Baumrind, 2013; Janssens, 1986; Maccoby & Martin, 1983). It is important to distinguish this form of behavioural control from psychological control. Psychological control involves control by parents through manipulative upbringing techniques such as guilt induction, shaming strategies, fear induction and conditional attention (Barber, 1996).

When signs of forthcoming problems arise, the transition is made to level two of vigilant care. Progression to this stage usually takes place when parents are presented with a slightly problematic situation, which is sometimes referred to as 'upbringing tension' (Burggraaff-Huiskes, 2007; Kousemaker & Timmers-Huigens, 1985). The problem behaviour is relatively limited and of recent occurrence and it concerns a parenting situation that no longer runs smoothly. Parents experience the behaviour in question as disagreeable and disappointing. They record their own mistakes and shortcomings. The situation causes slight stress (Burggraaff-Huiskes, 2007; Kousemaker & Timmers-Huigens, 1985).

In the face of this stress, parents tend to consult themselves and each other more intensively. They also consult people from their social network regarding suitable approaches and possible solutions. However, this social support is often inadequate. Therefore, a low level of curative support may be necessary (Burggraaff-Huiskes, 2007; Kousemaker & Timmers-Huigens, 1985). Omer (2011) and Shimshoni *et al* (2015) argue that this curative support can be realised by moving to a situation of 'focused supervision' in which parents increase their presence by collecting specific information about their child's activities and by checking whether previously formulated rules and agreements are being violated.

'Unilateral actions', the third level of NA, are necessary when problems persist or increase further and when the situation has progressed to become a problematic parenting situation. The parenting problems are serious and burdensome, and parents themselves can no longer find solutions. Assistance is needed (Burggraaff-Huiskes, 2007; Kousemaker & Timmers-Huigens, 1985).

This assistance can take the form of introducing technical or instrumental improvements, improving the parents' interpretation framework or increasing their well-being (Ruijssenaars *et al*, 2012). With unilateral actions consisting of training parents in de-escalation techniques, creating a network of supporters, relationship gestures and techniques aimed at providing resistance (including announcements, sit-ins, telephone round, parental visits, etc.), Omer (2011) explicitly chooses to make technical and instrumental improvements. Focused questioning and gathering information are no longer sufficient. In addition to gathering information (which happens both at level two and level three), parents are made more competent by learning new skills that increase their repertoire of action (Ruijssenaars *et al*, 2012).

Training in these skills should also result in improved well-being. After all, the goal is to increase parental presence, increase their experience of support and reduce parental helplessness (Omer, 2011). When we compare techniques and skills used within the framework of unilateral actions as used in NA with the techniques and skills used in NVR, it becomes clear that these are exactly the same techniques and resources. The third level of NA therefore corresponds to NVR (see Figure 7.1).

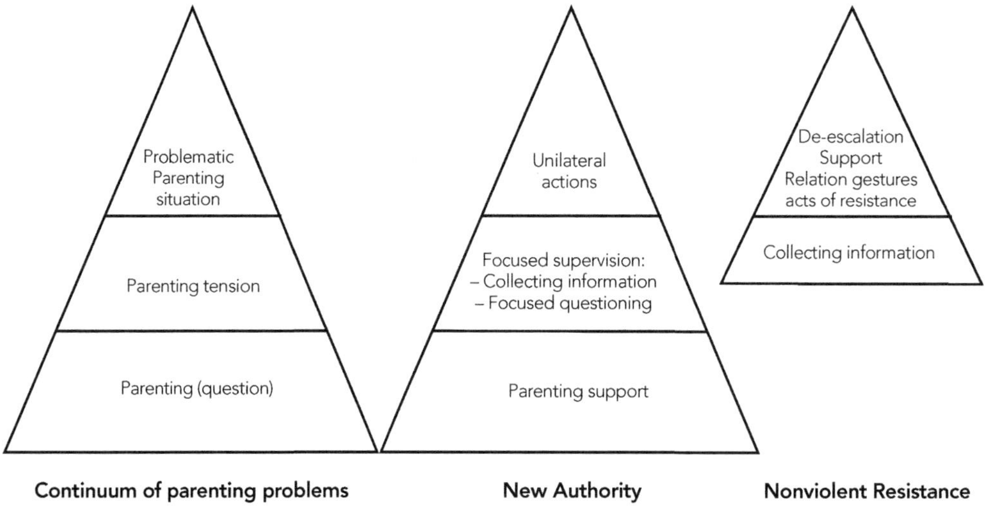


**Figure 7.1: NA and NVR in relation to a continuum of parenting problems**

# Five basic questions that characterise interventions

After having argued that we are indeed dealing with interventions embedded in a positive parenting climate, we focus on the five basic questions that characterise interventions. We do this mainly for NVR as an intervention as this has been examined the most and is best documented in the literature. We looked at sources beginning with the first publication in 1999 of the book *Parental Presence* (Omer, 1999) and ending with publications in 2016. We found a total of 98 references including 27 books and 71 articles in the English (36.7%), the German (32.7%) and the Dutch (30.6%) literature. There are 82 unique references and 16 translations. For an overview see www.bigv.be/literatuur/

## The target group: who is the intervention aimed at?

About 30% of the literature describes applications for specific target groups, which usually go hand in hand with adjustments to the needs and characteristics of the target group. There is an expansion from parents of children with violent and self-destructive behaviour (Omer, 2004) to parents of children/adolescents with ADHD (Jakob, 2014), with OCD (Lebowitz, 2013), with a psychotic disorder (Goddard *et al*, 2009), with anxiety disorders (Lebowitz *et al*, 2014), parents of children who use violence against siblings (Omer *et al*, 2008), those who refuse to go to school (Schorr-Sapir, 2011), who are addicted to the internet (Omer, 2011), who threaten suicide (Omer & Dolberger, 2015), and parents of young adults with autism (e.g. Golan *et al*, 2016) or adults who remain dependent on parents and make extreme demands (Lebowitz *et al*, 2012).

Although the intervention is often presented as an intervention for children and young people with specific problems, it is in fact aimed at parental figures who face coercive behaviour or behaviour that requires parental proximity and supervision (Omer & Lebowitz, 2016). Due to the problem behaviour, parents, family members and other parental figures become helpless and get the feeling that they have to adapt to these behaviours. The fact that the intervention targets parents or parental figures as clients is also manifest in applications for 'multi-stressed families' (Jakob, 2016), teachers (e.g. Omer, 2011), group educators (e.g. von Schlippe & Grabbe, 2007) and residents of problem quarters (Omer, 2011).

## What are its goals?

The original goals were numerous:

- helping parents in dealing with behavioural problems (e.g. Omer, 2001)
- reducing problem behaviour of children/youngsters (e.g. Omer, 2004)
- increasing the well-being of parents and support (e.g. Weinblatt & Omer, 2008)
- reducing parental helplessness (e.g. Ollefs *et al*, 2009).

And the goals are becoming more diverse. They have now expanded to teaching the staff in residential facilities to use fewer power resources (such as exclusion) (Amiel, 2011), supporting teachers to address problems in their class/school (e.g. Lemme *et al*, 2009) and helping local residents to reduce problem behaviour in their neighbourhood (e.g. Omer, 2011), among many others.

Core goals that always feature are a reduction in the sense of powerlessness and subjugation of authority figures. Training should result in an increased sense of self-esteem in the parenting figure. Parenting figures are taught to resist provocations (Omer, 2004; Weinblatt & Omer, 2008). Coercive cycles are broken and parenting figures no longer give in to unreasonable demands from youngsters (Omer & Dolberger, 2015). All this should result in parenting figures giving youngsters more structure, being more present, increasing their self-control and preventing escalations (Omer *et al*, 2013; Omer & Dolberger, 2015).

## Providers and application areas (who administers them?)

Treatment providers were initially therapists who work with parents with children with coercive behaviour. As NVR is a well-defined intervention (Omer *et al*, 2013), it can be applied by multiple professional groups in multiple domains. It is not intended that the intervention is solely conducted by certified therapists under the supervision of certified supervisors (Omer & Lebowitz, 2016). Meanwhile, the intervention is also used by family counsellors, foster care workers, residential care workers and others (Van Holen *et al*, 2011). These care workers work in their own practices, but also in specific contexts such as psychiatric wards (Goddard *et al*, 2009), residential facilities (e.g. Huybrechts, 2013), home guidance/crisis interventions at home (Van Holen *et al*, 2013), foster care (e.g. Vanschoonlandt *et al*, 2012), adoption (Van Moorter, 2015), education (e.g. Lemme *et al*, 2011) and, nurseries (Lipschitz, in Van Holen *et al*, 2011), the business world (Baumann-Habersack, 2015), and the broad community (e.g. Omer, 2011).

## What does the intervention consist of?

Although there is no strict protocol for the NVR programme (Lavi-Levavi *et al*, 2013; Omer & Dolberger, 2015), there are a number of techniques that can be called core techniques, namely: de-escalation training, creating a network of supporters, relationship gestures, and acts of resistance as the announcement, the sit-in, the documentation of aggressive behaviour, telephone round, parental visitations and acts of reparation (Lavi-Levavi *et al*, 2013; Omer & Dolberger, 2015; Omer & Lebowitz, 2016; Weinblatt & Omer, 2008). They all serve the same purposes: to increase parental presence, to help parents create structure for their child, to increase parental self-control and to increase social support. It is worth noting that the repertoire of the NVR therapist is expanding and/or worked out in depth. For example, Grabbe (2009) elaborated the concept of reconciliation to relationship gestures, Rodenburg and de Tempe (2015) describe difficulties concerning emotion regulation of traumatised parents, Weinblatt (2013) describes shame and shame regulation, and Jakob (2016) seeks solutions in the case of disqualifying networks, etc.

## Effectiveness (what does the intervention yield?)

We are now going to focus on what the literature tells us about both the effectiveness ('Does it work?') and intervention processes ('Why does(n't) it work?'). Note that all the studies below focus on the NVR programme, with the exception of Shimshoni *et al* (2015), which examines the NA framework.

### Effectiveness

Three factors are important in the evaluation of the effectiveness of interventions: statistical significance, clinical relevance and effect size. Statistical significance means that it is not likely that a difference between pre- and post-measurement has arisen by chance. A problem with statistical significance is that big differences in small samples are often statistically not significant, and that small differences in large samples can be significant while they are practically insignificant. Clinical relevancy is examined according to the number of clients for whom the risk/the disorder is gone, the problem is solved, or the situation returned to normal. Finally, the effect size is an indication of the extent of the effect. The effect size becomes increasingly important in research.

There are numerous case descriptions in literature (e.g. Omer, 2011; Omer *et al*, 2008; Omer & Dolberger, 2015) that illustrate interventions and adaptations to specific groups and contexts and that describe the therapeutic process and the techniques used. They document the challenges faced by clients and therapists and reflect the complexity of the therapeutic process. Numerous vignettes suggest that problem behaviours and violence between siblings decreases, helplessness of parents decreases, social support increases, etc. They form a first tentative indication that the intervention can be effective in the described issues and contexts.

Table 7.1 describes the results of six peer-reviewed articles (four from Israel, one from the United Kingdom and one from Belgium). They all concern research without a control group, based on self-report questionnaires, with pre- and post-measurements without follow-up, mostly in small and specific target groups. Three studies concern parents of children with OCD (Lebowitz, 2013), anxiety disorder (Lebowitz *et al*, 2014) or aggressive, violent and controlling behaviour (Newman *et al*, 2014). Van Holen *et al* (2016) describe a pilot with foster children with externalising problem behaviour.

In addition, two studies examine parents with resident (young) adults with autism (Golan *et al*, 2016) or who are highly dependent with extreme demands (Lebowitz *et al*, 2012). Mostly the interventions consist of 10 to 12 weekly sessions, with or without intermediate telephone support (Golan *et al*, 2016; Lebowitz, 2013; Lebowitz *et al*, 2014; Van Holen *et al*, 2016). Newman *et al* (2014) on the other hand, examined the effects of 12 group sessions with intermediate telephone support. Only Lebowitz *et al* (2012) deviate largely from the other interventions regarding the intensity by offering between 15 and 25 sessions.

The statistical significance of changes at group level was examined in all pilots. Only Van Holen *et al* (2016) also calculated effect sizes and examined the effects on an individual level. In general, all pilots suggest that problem behaviour and symptoms decrease, and that family functioning and the functioning of the parents improve. These non-controlled pilot studies form a second tentative indication that NVR can be effective for the described target populations. However, since no use was made of a control group, it cannot be shown that the effects are the result of the intervention.

## Table 7.1: Overview pilot studies

| Authors | Sample | Age N | Results | Treatment |
|---|---|---|---|---|
| Lebowitz, 2013 | Parents of children diagnosed OCD | 11-13 $n = 6$ | Significant decrease of:<br>■ OCD-symptoms<br>■ the need for adjustment by the family to these symptoms<br>■ disturbing and coercive behaviour. | 10 individual weekly sessions |
| Lebowitz *et al*, 2014 | Parents of children with anxiety disorder | 9-13 $n = 10$ | Significant decrease in anxiety symptoms and adjustment of the family to these symptoms.<br>Significant increase in the child's motivation for individual treatment. | 10 to 12 individual weekly sessions |

 

| Authors | Sample | Age N | Results | Treatment |
|---|---|---|---|---|
| Newman *et al*, 2014 | Parents of children with aggressive, violent and controlling behaviour | 8-17 *n* = 24 | Significant decrease of behaviour problems (although they remain clinical), and improved family functioning (parents handle behaviour better, quality of life is improved). | 12 bi-weekly group sessions with telephone support |
| Van Holen *et al*, 2016 | Foster parents of children with externalising problem behaviour | 6-18 *n* = 25 | On group level: significant decrease in problem behaviour in foster children: large effects on externalising and total problems, and medium effects on internalising behaviour problems.<br><br>Significant decrease in parental stress in foster parents (medium to large effect).<br><br>Individual: significant decrease externalising behaviour in 72%, internalising behaviour in 44% and total problems in 80%. In case of decrease, decrease was clinically significant in respectively 61.1%, 63.6% and 70%. | 10 individual weekly sessions with telephone support |
| Lebowitz *et al*, 2012 | Parents of highly dependent adults with extreme demands | 18-47 *n* = 46 | Significant decrease in usage of age-inappropriate services by parents; improvement in the functioning and in the employment of the adult children. | 15-25 individual sessions, initially weekly, subsequently spread |

| Authors | Sample | Age N | Results | Treatment |
|---|---|---|---|---|
| Golan *et al*, 2016 | Parents of young adults with high functioning autism | 20-26 $n = 4$ | Significant decrease in depression symptoms and increase of hope in parents. | 10 individual weekly sessions with telephone support |

The peer-reviewed articles listed in Table 7.2 (on page 103) describe five controlled trials (four randomised controlled trials (RCT) and one quasi-experimental study) in which an experimental group is compared with a control group (three from Israel, one from Germany and one from Belgium).

In a quasi-experimental research design with pre- and post-measurement without follow up, Ollefs *et al* (2009) compared a group of 48 mothers and 11 fathers who received NVR treatment (NVR group) with 18 mothers and three fathers who participated in teen triple P group training (PPP group), and a control group of six mothers and three fathers who received no training. They found a significant improvement in parental presence and parenting behaviour in both the NVR group and the PPP group compared to the control group. In addition, there was a significant decrease in depression symptoms in both the NVR group and the PPP group. Problem behaviour of the child improved significantly in the NVR group compared to both other groups. With regard to co-operation between parents, no effects were found. It cannot be determined, however, whether these effects were the result of the treatment. Indeed, a critical approach is warranted. First, by including both mothers and fathers, data were not independent. Second, the groups differed from each other regarding behavioural problems, depression, age and other variables, and these differences were not controlled.

In an RCT with pre- and post-measurement and one-month follow up, Weinblatt and Omer (2008) compared an NVR group of 21 families with 21 families on a waiting list. Significant decreases were found in levels of helplessness and permissive upbringing by the parents, and on problem behaviour in the children. Significant large effects with regard to support for mothers after treatment disappeared in follow up. No differences were found in parenting stress, authoritarian and authoritative parenting.

In an RCT with pre- and post-measurements and one-month follow up only in the experimental group, Lavi-Levavi, Shachar and Omer (2013) compared an NVR group of 26 families with a waiting list condition of 20 families. In this study, parents reported not only about themselves, but also about their partners. For both parents, there was a significant decrease of helplessness. According to the fathers only, there was also a significant decrease in power struggle, negative feelings and submission. Both parents agreed that the mother was worse off. Effect sizes were not calculated.

In an RCT with pre- and post-measurements and a three-month follow up, Van Holen *et al* (2016b) compared a sample of 31 foster families who received NVR with 31 foster families receiving care as usual. Significant medium-sized effects were found regarding the size of the supportive network (extension), significant medium-sized effects regarding parenting stress (decrease), and small to medium (positive) effects regarding some parenting behaviours. With regard to behaviour problems in foster children, only small non-significant decreases were found.

Shimshoni *et al* (2015) examined the effects of one NVR session aimed at increasing vigilant care by parents and feedback on the driving behaviour of young drivers, with the addition of a punishment. This intervention had a significant positive impact on driving behaviour.

The studies in Table 7.2 show that NVR is effective and can lead to a decrease of problem behaviours in children, adolescents and young people (between four and 21 years), a decrease in parental feelings of helplessness and stress, and an extension of the supportive network of foster parents. The research of Shimshoni *et al* (2015) shows that NA can also have preventive effects. This can inspire to develop and examine other preventive interventions.

However, there are still many uncertainties and many questions remain unanswered. We focus on them in the process evaluation.

## Table 7.2: Controlled trials

| Study | Sample | Design | Results | Treatment |
|---|---|---|---|---|
| Ollefs *et al*, 2009 | 89 parents with children with externalising problem behaviour | Quasi-experimental: **NVR:** 48 mothers, 11 fathers<br>**Teen-Triple P:** 18 mothers, 3 fathers<br>**Control:** 6 mothers, 3 fathers<br>Pre, post, no follow-up<br>Self-report | Significant favourable changes (no effect sizes calculated) regarding parental presence, parenting behaviour and depression in parents and significant decrease in problem behaviour.<br>No improvements in the collaboration between parents. | ?? sessions,<br>?? telephone support |

| Study | Sample | Design | Results | Treatment |
|---|---|---|---|---|
| Weinblatt, & Omer, 2008 | 41 middleclass families with children (4-17 years) with externalising problem behaviour | RCT<br>(21 exp.–21 control)<br>Pre, post, follow up 1 month<br>Self-report | Significant decreases in helplessness and permissive education in the parents and problem behaviour in the children (mainly by mothers).<br>No permanent effects on support, no effects on authoritarian and authoritative education. | 5-10 individual sessions with telephone support |
| Lavi-Levavi *et al*, 2013 | 46 two-parent middleclass families with children with acute externalising problem behaviour | RCT<br>(26 exp.–20 control)<br>Pre, post, follow-up of 1 month only in the exp. group<br>Reporting about himself and about partner | Significant changes (no effect sizes calculated) in helplessness (decrease) both within themselves as within their partner.<br>According to fathers only, significant decrease in power struggles, negative feelings and submission.<br>According to both, mothers are worse off. | 4-10 individual sessions, with telephone support (2x/ week) |
| Van Holen, *et al*, 2016b | Foster mothers with a foster child (6-18 years) with externalising problem behaviour | RCT<br>(31 exp–31 control)<br>Pre, post, follow-up 3 months<br>Self-report | Significant medium effects on the size of the supporting network, significant medium effects on parenting stress (decrease) and small to medium sized (positive) effects on some parenting behaviours.<br>Only small effects (decrease) on behavioural problems. | 10 individual sessions with telephone support |

 

| Study | Sample | Design | Results | Treatment |
|---|---|---|---|---|
| Shimshoni *et al*, 2015 | Young drivers (17–22 years) | Individual feedback (*n*=49)<br>Family feedback (*n*=52)<br>Vigilant care (*n*=52) | Significant positive influence on the driving behaviour of youngsters | 1 session |

## Process evaluation

A process evaluation aims to figure out in a systematic way what works and what doesn't (Lipsey & Cordray, 2000). Process evaluations are becoming increasingly important because they help to understand the results of effectiveness evaluations, and form the basis for improvement (e.g. Bartholomew *et al*, 2011; Saunders *et al*, 2005). Roughly speaking, there are two different forms of process evaluations:

- Development, functioning and effectuation: examines what has gone well and what hasn't, if the approach is feasible and works as intended.
- Appreciation and experience of performers and participants: examines what it means to them, if they are satisfied, and whether the intervention delivers what they expect.

There are however few guidelines for carrying out process evaluations (Saunders *et al*, 2005). Furthermore, process evaluations are often not published, or at least not systematically published. Saunders *et al* (2005) developed a model to conduct process evaluations in which they distinguished four components that need to be ascertained: (1) recruitment and range, (2) faithfulness of implementation, (3) dose and satisfaction, and (4) context. Below, for the four controlled NVR trials, we describe what is documented on these four components.

### Recruitment and range

The central question here is how many and which participants were reached. However, the cited research is not always clear on the characteristics of the participants and a lot of fog remains. The ages of the children of the included families is only clearly reported by Weinblatt and Omer (2008) and Van Holen *et al* (2016). They respectively included (foster) families with (foster) children aged four to 18 and six to 18 years. Lavi-Levavi *et al* (2013) included families with children up to 18 years but don't report on the lower limit, while Ollefs *et al* (2009) don't mention the ages of the children at all. This leaves it unclear whether NVR also works in (foster) families with very young children.

Concerning the socio-economic status of the families, Weinblatt and Omer (2008) and Lavi-Levavi *et al* (2009) studied middleclass families while Van Holen, Vanderfaeillie *et al* (2016) also included foster families with low socio-economic background. Ollefs *et al* (2009) don't report on this characteristic. Therefore, the effectiveness of NVR interventions in families from different socio-economic classes remains unclear.

Weinblatt and Omer (2008) and Lavi-Levavi *et al* (2013) included families with children with acute problem behaviour, while Ollefs *et al* (2009) and Van Holen *et al* (2016) included (foster) children with chronic problem behaviour, although it remains unclear for how long. Van Holen *et al* (2016) only included foster families with foster children who had a borderline or clinical score on the externalising problem scale of the Child Behavior Checklist (Achenbach & Rescorla, 2001), while in the other studies it remains unclear whether included children had clinical scores. This leaves it unclear as to whether NVR is as effective with families with children with chronic behaviour problems as it is with those with acute problem behaviours, and whether it as effective with families with children with many problem behaviours as it is with children who have few problem behaviours.

Problems faced by families were neither reported nor compared with standard data, which leaves it unclear how helpless parents were and how deviant their parental stress and parental behaviours were.

## Faithfulness of implementation

The fidelity of the interventions to the principles of NVR, and the quality of their implementation are essential to be able to judge their effectiveness (Saunders *et al*, 2005). To do this, we examined the extent to which core components of the interventions were delivered as prescribed (Nelson *et al*, 2012). Only Van Holen *et al* (2016) report on the use of treatment checklists and bi-weekly supervision sessions aimed at protecting treatment fidelity. In the other studies it remains unclear to what extent the therapeutic protocol was followed.

The core components of NVR as already described, are: (1) de-escalation training, (2) support, (3) reconciliation gestures and (4) resistance against problem behaviour. Three of the studies reported the extent to which core components of NVR were used by the (foster) families. These are shown in Table 7.3.

 

The core components were used by the large majority of the (foster) families involved in these three studies. There were notable differences in the use of different acts of resistance against problem behaviour, where announcements were used by almost all the families but the use of other acts varied widely. This can partly be explained by the fact that some actions are used to address specific problem behaviours (e.g. a telephone round when a child doesn't come home or gets home too late), but other reasons, such as resistance of the therapist or the parents, or cultural differences, cannot be ruled out.

## Table 7.3: Implemented core components/actions

| Core components/actions | Weinblatt & Omer (2008) | Ollefs (2008) | Van Holen (2014) |
|---|---|---|---|
| De-escalation | 100 | 100 | 100 |
| Resistance – increase parental presence | 100 | 98 | 100 |
| Announcement | 100 | 98 | 100 |
| Visitation – telephone round | 90 | 10 | 65 |
| Sit-in | 65 | 2 | 26 |
| Reparation act | unknown | unknown | 26 |
| Documentation of aggressive behaviour | unknown | unknown | 23 |
| Refusal of services | unknown | 2 | unknown |
| Reconciliation – relation gestures | 100 | 100 | 100 |
| Support | 90 | 96 | 84 |

## Dose and satisfaction

In this section, three aspects are distinguished: the amount of treatment delivered by the therapist, the amount of treatment received by the participants, and the satisfaction of participants. The amount of treatment is very much linked with the fidelity of implementation, as discussed in the previous section.

Only Van Holen (2014) reports on client satisfaction using the BESTE – Rating Scale Satisfaction and Effect[2] (De Meyer *et al*, 2004). Both foster parents and regular foster care workers were surveyed and table 7.4 gives an overview of the percentage of foster mothers and foster care workers who responded affirmative to questions.

2 'Beoordelingsschaal Tevredenheid en Effect'

The large majority of both foster mothers and foster care workers reported that the intervention contributed to a decrease in behavioural problems in the foster child, improved family functioning, improved parenting, and a better understanding of the behaviour of the foster child. It is not surprising that almost all foster mothers and foster care workers would recommend the intervention to others.

## Table 7.4: Client satisfaction

| BESTE (question) | Foster mothers (% reporting improvement) | Foster care worker (% reporting improvement) |
|---|---|---|
| Has the behaviour of your foster child changed? | 82.1 | 80.6 |
| Has something changed in the functioning of your family? | 96.6 | 87.1 |
| Has something changed in the way you educate your foster child? | 93.1 | 86.7 |
| Has your view of your foster child's behaviour been clarified? | 85.2 | 93.5 |
| Would you recommend the intervention to others? | 96.3 | 93.6 |

Regarding the duration of the intervention, there was less unanimity and while the majority of foster mothers and foster care workers indicated that the intervention lasted exactly long enough, an important group of foster mothers and foster care workers indicated that the duration was too short.

## Table 7.5: Satisfaction regarding the duration of the intervention

| Duration | Foster mothers | Foster care workers |
|---|---|---|
| Too short | 32 | 35.7 |
| Exactly long enough | 68 | 57.1 |
| Too long | 0 | 7.1 |

Another indication of satisfaction is dropout rate, which was reported by three of the studies:

- Weinblatt & Omer (2008): one family (4.8%) from the experimental group dropped out prematurely.
- Lavi-Levavi *et al* (2013): reported the drop-out of two families (7.7%)
- Van Holen *et al* (2016): no families (0%).

These percentages are remarkably low – after all, drop-outs are a problem in most parent training programmes (Friars & Mellor, 2009). Forehand *et al* (1983) report in their review a drop-out percentage of 28%. Other estimates range from 30% to 60% (Baekeland & Lundwall; in Friars & Mellor, 2007).

### Context

Context focuses on possible changes in the organisation or in the broader context during the research period (Linnan & Steckler, 2002) but none of the studies reported on this. Nevertheless, Van Holen *et al* (2015) investigated the support offered to the control group by comparing the treatment-as-usual that was offered to the control group with treatment-as-usual that was offered to a matched group of foster parents who did not participate in the RTC. The results show that being assigned to the control group had a significant effect on the support that foster parents received and was associated with both a significantly higher support frequency offered by the foster care worker, and with significantly more referrals to and service use for both foster parents and foster children. Consequently, the control group received enhanced treatment as usual, which may have affected the results unfavourably.

## Conclusion

Since 1999, the concepts NVR, NA and Vigilant Care have increasingly entered into counselling and research literature. There is an evolution from a manualised family therapeutic *curative* intervention aimed at reducing problem behaviour (NVR), to a broader pedagogical framework that can be used both *preventively* and *curatively* by all parental figures that may or may not be confronted with coercive behaviour or behaviour that requires parental presence and supervision (NA).

In this chapter we focused on five questions that characterise interventions. Special attention was given to the effectiveness of NVR. Numerous case descriptions and six pilot studies suggest that NVR might be effective for specific target populations. Nevertheless, only four peer-reviewed controlled studies were published. They indicate that NVR is effective and results in:

- a decrease of problem behaviour in children and youngsters (between four and 21 years).

- a decrease in the helplessness felt by parents and parental stress in both natural parents and foster parents.
- an extension of the supportive network of foster parents.

We conclude that NVR and NA are therefore 'more than a good idea'. Nevertheless, research is lagging well behind the increase of the target groups and the application areas. Currently, according to the criteria of Chambless and Hollon (1998), the most that can be decided is that NVR is 'probably (an) effective' intervention. Although there are four control studies in which an NVR-group was compared with a control group, the follow-up periods were short (one to three months) or non-existent, the examined samples were small and only two studies reported effect sizes. In addition, Omer is always a (co-)author, therefore the independence of the studies is questionable. In regard to preventive programmes, empirical evidence for their efficacy remains scarce. Up to now, only one control study has been described.

In addition, there is a lack of systematic process evaluations that can provide more insight into which elements of the intervention are effective and what can or should be improved. The core components of the intervention were implemented to a large extent in all four studies, but differences exist regarding the use of specific actions. Low drop-out rates and high satisfaction rates suggest that the intervention is positively honoured by parents.

Nevertheless, many questions and uncertainties remain and will determine the future research agenda. In particular, rigorous research with multi-trait, multi-method research designs in a wide range of application areas is needed with a clear description of the problem and of the characteristics of both the parental figures and their children, adolescents and young adults. Furthermore, what actions/elements are essential, and their relative effectiveness, should be examined over a longer period of time, as well as the optimal duration of the treatment. To date, only the experiences of the (foster) parents were examined. Future research should focus on experiences of children and young people too.

NVR is a promising intervention. Empirical evidence and scientific underpinning is increasing but lags far behind the rapid development of the ideas and a broadening of the goals, target groups and the target areas of the intervention. There is an urgent need for more thorough research on the effectiveness of NVR and NA in order to define the possibilities and the limits of this intervention more clearly.

 

# References

Achenbach TM & Rescorla LA (2001) *Manual for the Aseba school-age forms and profiles: Child behavior checklist for ages 6-18.* Burlington: ASEBA.

Amiel I (2011) NVR implementations in a closed ward. In: F Van Holen, A Lampo, and J Vanderfaeillie (Eds.) *Applications and Illustrations of Nonviolent Resistance and New Authority in Family Therapy, Education and Psychiatric Care* (pp73–78). Brussels: VUBPRESS.

Barber BK (1996) Parental psychological control: revisiting a neglected construct. *Child Development* 67 3296–3319.

Bartholomew KL, Parcel GS, Kok G & Gottlieb NH (2011). *Planning health promotion programs: An intervention mapping approach* (3rd ed.). San Francisco: Jossey-Bass.

Baumann-Habersack F (2015) *Mit neuer Autorität in Führung. Warum wir heute präsenter, beharrlicher und vernetzter führen müssen.* Heidelberg: Springer Gabler.

Baumrind D (1971) Current patterns of parental authority. *Development Psychology Monograph* **4** 1–103.

Baumrind D (2013) Is a pejorative view of power assertion in the socialization process justified? *Review of General Psychology* **17** 420–427.

Bom H & Wiebenga E (2017) Verbindend gezag. Naar een nieuwe vorm van autoriteit gebaseerd op principes van geweldloos verzet. *Tijdschrift voor Psychotherapie* DOI 10.1007/s12485-017-0206-8.

Burggraaff-Huiskes M (2007) *Opvoedingsondersteuning als bijzondere vorm van preventie.* Bussum: Uitgeverij Coutinho.

Chambless DL & Hollon SD (1998) Defining empirically supported therapies. *Journal of Consulting and Clinical Psychology* **66** 7–18.

De Meyer RE, Janssen J & Veerman JW (2004) *Handleiding beoordelingsschaal tevredenheid en effect* (BESTE). Nijmegen: Praktikon.

Forehand R, Middlebrook J, Rogers T & Steffe M (1983) Dropping out of parent training. *Behavior Research and Therapy* **21** 663–668.

Friars P & Mellor D (2009) Drop-out from parenting training programmes: A retrospective study. *Journal of Child and Adolescent Mental Health* **21** 29–38.

Friars PM & Mellor DJ (2007) Drop out from behavioural management programs for ADHD: A prospective study. *Journal of Child and Family Studies* **16** 427–441.

Goddard N, Van Gink K, Van der Stegen B, Van Driel J & Cohen AP (2009) 'Smeed het ijzer als het koud is'. Non-Violent Resistance op een acuut psychiatrische afdeling voor adolescenten. *Maandblad Geestelijke Volksgezondheid* **64** 531–539.

Golan O, Shilo H & Omer H (2016) Non-violent resistance parent training for the parents of young adults with high functioning autism spectrum disorder. *Journal of Family Therapy* doi:10.1111/1467-6427.12106.

Grabbe M (2009) Es gibt keinen weg zu einer guten Beziehung – eine gute Beziehung ist der Weg. Bündnisrhetorik und praktische Beziehungsgestaltung von Eltern mit ihren Kindern. *Familiendynamik*, 34/3, 266–274.

Huybrechts A (2013) Waakzame zorg welkom in de residentiële context. *Systeemtheoretisch bulletin* **31** 49–65.

Jakob P (2014) Non-violent resistance and ADHD. *ADHD in Practice* **6** (2) 7–11.

Jakob P (2016) Multi-stressed Families, Child Violence and the Larger System: an Adaptation of the Nonviolent Model. *Journal of Family Therapy* doi: 10.1111/1467-6427.12133.

Janssens JMAM (1986) Opvoeding en ontwikkeling van kinderen. In: R De Groot and J van Weelden (Eds.) *Van Gisteren Over Morgen* (pp9–35). Groningen: Wolters-Noordhoff.

Kousemaker NPJ & Timmers-Huigens D (1985) Pedagogische hulpverlening in de eerste lijn. *Tijdschrift Voor Orthopedagogiek* **24** 549–565.

Lamborn SD, Mounts NS, Steinberg L & Dornbusch SM (1991) Patterns of Competence and adjustment among Adolescents from Authoritative, Authoritarian, Indulgent, and Neglectful Families. *Child Development* **62** 1049–1065.

Lavi-Levavi I, Shachar I & Omer H (2013) Training in nonviolent resistance for parents of violent children: differences between fathers and mothers. *Journal of Systemic Therapies* **32** (4) 79–93.

Lebowitz ER (2013) Parent-based treatment for children and adolescent OCD. *Journal of Obsessive-Compulsive and Related Disorders* **2** 425–431.

Lebowitz E, Dolberger D, Nortov E & Omer H (2012) Parent Training in Non Violent Resistance for Adult Entitled Dependence. *Family Process* **51** 90–106.

Lebowitz E, Omer H, Hermes H & Scahill L (2014) Parent Training for Childhood Anxiety Disorders: The SPACE Program. *Cognitive and Behavioral Practice* **21** 456–469.

Lemme M, Bojarzin R & Tepaße F (2011) Autorität durch Beziehung in der Schule. *Zeitschrift für Systemische Therapie und Beratung* **29** (2) 62–72.

Lemme M, Tillner R & Eberding A (2009) Neue Autorität in der Schule. *Familiendynamik* **34** (3) 276–283.

Linnan L & Steckler A (2002) Process Evaluation for Public Health Interventions and Research: An overview. In: A Stecklers and L Linnan (Eds.) *Process Evaluation for Public Health Interventions and Research* (pp1-23). San Francisco: Jossey-Bass.

Lipsey MW & Cordray DS (2000) Evaluation methods for social intervention. *Annual Review of Psychology* **51** 345–375.

Lipschitz N (2011) Reparation acts – NVR in kindergartens. In: F Van Holen, A Lampo & J Vanderfaeillie (Eds.) *Applications and Illustrations of Nonviolent Resistance and New Authority in Family Therapy, Education and Psychiatric Care* (pp51–57). Brussels: VUBPRESS.

Maccoby EE & Martin JA (1983) Socialization in the context of the family: parent-child interaction. In: PH Mussen and ME Hetherington (Eds.) *Handbook of Child Psychology: Vol. 4. Socialization, personality, and social development* (pp1–101). New York: Wiley.

Nelson MC, Cordray DS, Hulleman CS, Darrow CL & Sommer EC (2012) A procedure for assessing intervention fidelity in experiments testing educational and behavioural interventions. *Journal of Behavioral Health Services and Research*, **39** (4) 1–22.

Newman M, Fagan C & Webb R (2014) The efficacy of non-violent resistance groups in treating aggressive and controlling behaviour in children and young people: a preliminary analysis of pilot NVR groups in Kent. *Child and Adolescent Mental Health* **19** (2) 138–141.

Ollefs B (2008) *Jugendliche mit externalem problemverhalten. Effekte von elterncoaching.* Doctoral Dissertation, Humanwissenschaften, Universität Osnabrück.

Ollefs B, von Schlippe A, Omer H & Kriz J (2009) Jugendliche mit externalem Problemverhalten. Effekte von Elterncoaching. *Familiendynamik* **34** 3 256–265.

Omer H (1999) Parental presence. *Reclaiming a leadership role in bringing up our children.* Phoenix Arizona: Zeig, Tucker and Co.

Omer H (2001) Helping parents deal with children's acute disciplinary problems without escalation: the principle of non-violent resistance. *Family Process* **40** 1 53–66.

 

Omer H (2004) *Nonviolent Resistance. A new approach to violent and self-destructive children*. New York: Cambridge University Press.

Omer H (2011) *The New Authority: Family, school and community*. New York: Cambridge University Press.

Omer H & Dolberger D (2015) Helping parents cope with suicide threats: An approach based on nonviolent resistance. *Family Process* doi: 10.1111/famp.12129.

Omer H & Lebowitz E (2016) Nonviolent Resistance. Helping caregivers reduce problematic behaviors in children and adolescents. *Journal of Marital and Family Therapy* doi: 10.1111/jmft.12168.

Omer H, Satran S & Driter O (2017) Vigilant care: An integrative reformulation regarding parental monitoring. *Psychological Review* **123** (3) 291–304.

Omer H, Schorr-Sapir I & Weinblatt U (2008) Non-violent resistance and violence against siblings. *Journal of Family Therapy* **30** (4) 450–464.

Omer H, Steinmetz S, Carthy T & von Schlippe A (2013) The Anchoring Function: Parental authority and the parent-child bond. *Family Process* **52** 193–206.

Rodenburg L & de Tempe J (2015) Ik ben mijn kind spuugzat. Ouderlijke emotieregulatie en nieuwe autoriteit. *Systeemtherapie* **27** (2) 65–81.

Ruijssenaars AJJM, Van de Bergh PM & Van Drenth JML (2012) *Orthopedagogiek. Ontwikkelingen, theorieën en modellen*. Antwerpen/Apeldoorn: Garant.

Saunders RP, Evans MH & Joshi P (2005) Developing a process-evaluation plan for assessing health promotion program implementation: A how-to Guide. *Health Promotion Practice* **6** (2) 134–147.

Schorr-Sapir I (2011) School refusal. In: F Van Holen, A Lampo & J Vanderfaeillie (Eds.) *Applications and illustrations of nonviolent resistance and new authority in family therapy, education and psychiatric care* (pp61–66). Brussels: VUBPRESS.

Shachar-Lavi I (2011) Vigilant care. In: F Van Holen, A Lampo & J Vanderfaeillie (Eds.) *Applications and illustrations of nonviolent resistance and new authority in family therapy, education and psychiatric care* (pp21–26). Brussels: VUBPRESS.

Shimshoni Y, Farah H, Lotan T, Grimberg E, Dritter O, Musicant O, Toledo T & Omer H (2015) Effects of parental vigilant care and feedback on novice driver risk. *Journal of Adolescence* **38** 69–80.

Vanderfaeillie J & Van Holen F (2010) Het verloop van pleeggezinplaatsingen. In: P van den Bergh and T Weterings (Eds.) *Pleegzorg in perspectief. Ontwikkelingen in theorie en praktijk* (pp177–193). Assen: Van Gorcem.

Van Holen F (2014) *Ontwikkeling en implementatie van een trainingsprogramma voor pleegouders gebaseerd op Geweldloos Verzet*. Doctoral Dissertation, Brussel: VUB Press.

Van Holen F, Geens B & Vanderfaeillie J (2013) Empowerment van gezinnen vanuit 'non-violent resistance'. Ervaringen vanuit de werkvormen thuisbegeleiding en crisishulp aan huis. In: K De Corte, S Bal, I Antrop & E Van den Haute (Ed) *Empowerment van de context: een net van steun en stimulatie voor kwetsbare en gekwetste kinderen* (pp91–108). Apeldoorn: Garant.

Van Holen F, Lampo A & Vanderfaeillie J (Eds) (2011) *Applications and Illustrations of Non-Violent Resistance and the New Authority in Family Therapy, Education and Psychiatric Care*. Brussels: University Press.

Van Holen F, Vanderfaeillie J, De Maeyer S & Gypen L (2015) Does allocation to a control condition in a Randomized Controlled Trial affect the routine care foster parents receive? *Children and Youth Services Review* **49** 48–53.

Van Holen F, Vanderfaeillie J & Omer H (2016a) Adaptation and evaluation of a nonviolent resistance intervention for foster parents: A progress report. *Journal of Marital and Family Therapy* **42** (2) 256–271.

Van Holen F, Vanderfaeillie J, Omer H & Vanschoonlandt F (2016b) Training in nonviolent resistance for foster parents: a randomized controlled trial. *Research on Social Work Practice* DOI: 10.1177/1049731516662915.

Van Moorter H (2015) Zoektocht naar herstel: een zoon en zijn adoptieouders samen op weg. *Systeemtheoretisch Bulletin* **33** 109–122.

Vanschoonlandt F, Van Holen F & Vanderfaeillie J (2012) Ontwikkeling en proefimplementatie van twee ondersteuningsprogramma's voor pleegouders. *Orthopedagogiek: Onderzoek en Praktijk* **51** 69–83.

Van Yperen T, Roosma D & Veerman JW (2008) Instrumenten voor het meten van uitkomsten en uitvoering van de zorg. In: T van Yperen and JW Veerman (Eds.), *Zicht op effectiviteit. Handboek voor praktijkgericht effectonderzoek in de jeugdzorg*. (pp245–270). Delft: Eburon.

von Schlippe A & Grabbe M (2007) *Werkstattbuch Elterncoaching. Elterliche Präsenz und gewaltloser Widerstand in der Praxis.* Göttingen: Vandenhoeck and Ruprecht.

Weinblatt U (2013) Die Regulierung des Schamgefühls bei intensive Eltern-Kind-Konflikten. Praktiken des gewaltlosen Widerstands, die die Öffentlichkeit einbeziehen. *Familiëndynamik* **38** 62–71.

Weinblatt U & Omer H (2008) Nonviolent resistance: a treatment for parents of children with acute behaviour problems. *Journal of Marital and Family Therapy* **34** 75–92.

Wells K (1997) The death of discipline: is the requiem premature? *Aggression and Violent Behavior* **2** 337–341.

 

# Part 2: Working for a better future

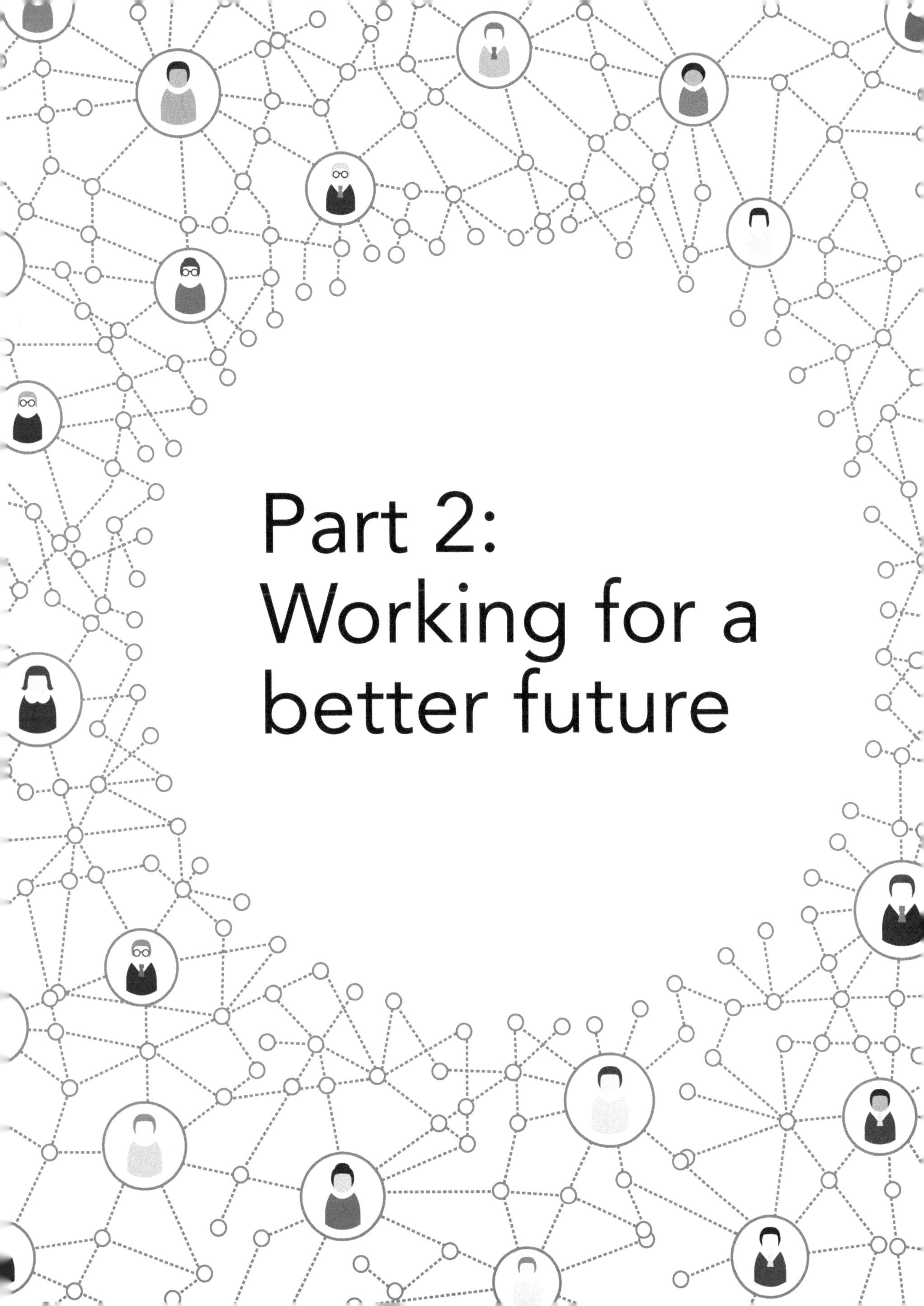

# Chapter 8: Building trust and co-operation between Israel police and Israeli-Arab citizens

**By Ziv Gilad, PhD – translated from the Hebrew by Carmit Gilad**

## Introduction

Israel police and Israeli-Arab citizens have experienced many violent and costly conflicts, leading to hatred, hostility and mistrust.

Police officers are traditionally seen in Arabic society as prominent representatives of old-school authority. They are granted significant powers and demand unconditional obedience, while meting out harsh punishments. The police are also used as cultural symbols of abuse of authority. The image of the cruel, oppressive policeman who humiliates those under his control is one of the major obstacles to police activity in the Arab sector.

In recent years, the Israeli police have been advancing activities designed to rebuild trust and establish better co-operation with Arab citizens, aiming to reduce crime and strengthen civilians' sense of personal safety. This has been done in the spirit of NVR, or 'connecting authority'.

When following these connecting authority principles, police officers are not called into action only as a last resort, but rather are regular partners in the ongoing struggle against crime. They are no longer expected to show up, intimidate and overpower; nor are they expected to do all the work where others have failed. Now, police officers represent an authority that draws on being part of a social system. Results are achieved when police and the community network are mutually strengthened by each other's influence.

This chapter describes and illustrates how implementing the principles of non-violent resistance has reduced resentment of the police among Israeli-Arab citizens; contributed to the development of trust; and helped create a network of community leaders, local authority officials and the police, all working together to minimise crime within the Arab sector.

## Policing in the Arab Sector in Israel

Ever since its creation, the state of Israel has experienced violent conflicts with its neighbouring Arab countries, as well as with the Israeli-Arab/Palestinian population within the country itself[3]. The political disagreement between the Jewish and Arab sectors has a significant impact on the interaction between Israeli Arabs and the police. The Arab minority is indigenous, with its own language and culture, and little desire to assimilate in Jewish society, nor does the Jewish majority wish to have them assimilated (Harpaz, 2008). Complaints from Arab society about injustice and inequality from governmental authorities have brought about a general objection to police work in Arab neighbourhoods (Santo & Ali, 2008; Hasisi, 2016).

Until recently, Arab society has not been a high priority of the government, police and other law enforcement bodies. This seems to have created a tendency to ignore crimes occurring within Arab towns or villages. The Arab population, in turn, has not been co-operating with the police, and civilians have tended to avoid filing complaints about relatives or neighbours, particularly in cases of violent assaults, because, as some argue, they mistrust the police and law enforcement officials and feel they should have autonomy in managing these offenses (Ali, 2014).

The Jewish population in Israel also express racist sentiments including stereotypes, distrust, rejection and various forms of discrimination. One survey (Harpaz, 2008) that examined attitudes among Jewish Israelis toward the Arab population found that 55% of the Jewish citizens view Israeli-Arabs as a security danger. Some Jews see the Arabs as 'primitive' and incapable of reaching their own level of development (Harpaz, 2008).

Considering that in many countries police attitudes tend to reflect the cultural norms of the majority group, it is to be expected that there is a degree of distance and alienation between Israeli Arabs and the police. And this is cyclical, reinforcing the stereotypes on both sides and exacerbating the tensions between the police force and Arab civilians (Gofer & Ben porat, 2013).

3 This refers to Arabs/Palestinians (Muslims or Christians) who are Israeli citizens, as opposed to those living in the Palestinian Authority.

 

It is therefore important that Israeli police officers working in the Arab community exercise their authority in a way that will not distance them from the community but connect them to it. Improving relationships and increasing trust and co-operation between the police and Israeli-Arab citizens will significantly achieve this and benefit both sides. The ability of the police to apply authority in an effective and legitimate way, especially with minority groups, depends on those groups' trust in the police force. Having a fair and effective police force is essential to the daily lives of minorities (Samocha, 2005)

In recent years, the police have been putting great effort into changing its relations with the Israeli-Arab population. Several police stations have been established in Arab towns and villages to improve the service in those communities, and the community policing approach has been expanded, aiming to create trust and collaboration between police and residents. Despite these efforts, the nature of the job, the history of violent confrontations, and the inherited traditional image of the police in the eyes of Arab citizens have been significant obstacles to change.

Part of the challenge is the lack of an alternative image to this traditional one. The need for a different police image is one example of the broader social need for an image of authority that fits the values of a democratic society. In working with Arab police officers and civilians, I have found that the principles of 'connecting authority' (Bom & Wiebenga, 2017), based on the 'new authority model' (Omer, 2011), are acceptable to both sides as an organising model for their relationship. The next section elaborates on connecting authority and illustrates how it serves the police in its work with the Arab population.

## The connecting authority approach

Over the past few decades there has been a change in the authority of parents, teachers, police and other authority figures. While in the 1970s the 'old authority' was well-established, appreciated and accepted without question, today a traditionally authoritative role itself does not necessarily grant its owner – the police in this case – authority in the eyes of the public (Omer, 2011; Gilad, 2013). The 'old authority' was based on a police officer's demand for obedience, an emotional distance between them and the people they policed, an immediate, sometimes aggressive reaction to disobedience, and an attitude that held the civilian responsible for any escalation in the interaction.

Social changes, such as a growing emphasis on civil rights, public protest and the failure of the old authority to engender trust and co-operation with civilians, led to an inevitable shift in the perception of police authority, as well as other authority figures in the community. Now, police officers are required to do more to gain compliance, respect and co-operation. They need a 'new authority', better suited to contemporary thinking – in the form of 'connecting authority'.

# What is connecting authority?

To explain the connecting authority approach, I will focus on two policing areas: 1) routine presence, and 2) conflict management.

## Routine presence: from keeping a distance to being present

In the 'old authority' approach, the distance between police and civilians was important, and the police officer was supposed to always remain remote and firm. Today, civilians no longer accept this attitude – they know their rights, they feel equal, and they demand fairness and good service. Thus, the police have had to decrease distance and convey presence.

### What is the meaning of presence?

Showing presence means demonstrating care and concern for civilians' safety, while maintaining the basic distinction between police duties and civilians' responsibilities.

Many Israeli-Arab citizens expect the police to show sensitivity and concern toward their distresses and to act with determination to protect residents from criminal activities. The more the police become part of the community fabric – not just in response to emergency calls but in daily life in general – the more trust and closeness can be established and can replace suspicion, resentment and fear based on past events and stereotypes. This kind of contact can increase the rate at which civilians' report crime as they have more confidence that the police will respond effectively and appropriately.

## Conflict management

There are several crucial differences between a police officer's actions while following the guidelines of old authority, and his/her actions in the spirit of connecting authority. These differences are manifested in various areas, as shown in table 8.1.

 

## Table 8.1: Old vs. new authority

| Area | Old authority | Connecting authority |
|---|---|---|
| Use of force | Loud or violent interactions are caused by civilians; the policeman only reacts with force against force.<br><br>The police officer educates the civilian, and his/her use of force is justified.<br><br>In the context of the Israeli-Arab sector, which is perceived as dangerous and violent, the only way is to overpower and to intimidate. | Using force is the last resort, and the burden of proof is on the police officer.<br><br>An unjustified use of force is destructive to both sides; the police officer puts his/her job at risk and damages the police's public image. |
| The concept of respect | Any disrespect calls for a strong reaction.<br><br>Due to political and religious factors related to the conflict between the Israeli police and the Arab community, any resistance to police action is perceived as a challenge to the state and its symbols. | Police officers are faced with daily acts of disrespect and are aspiring to have the personal strength to keep events from escalating.<br><br>Policemen's source of power and pride lies in their ability to deal with conflicts calmly, and to negotiate rather than apply force. |
| Support from other organisations | The police officer is an exclusive authority and functions independently of the rest of the community. | The police officer is part of an internal and external organisational network that incorporates authority figures from different areas of the community to achieve common goals. |
| Constancy | No long-term thinking; focusing on the event at hand in an immediate and final manner.<br><br>No willingness or interest in acting continually within Arab communities. | Constancy and persistence are key principles. Police presence, not just at events, deters negative activities significantly and creates a sense of protection. |

| Area | Old authority | Connecting authority |
|---|---|---|
| Transparency and publicity | Policemen operate under a shield of confidentiality and are not expected to justify their use of authority.<br><br>Due to suspicion and secrecy, authority figures rely on themselves alone, particularly with regard to the Arab sector, which is perceived as distrustful and as undermining the government and state security. | Transparency and publicity are fundamental expectations in modern society and are used as an opportunity to publicise successful cases of conflict resolution and problem solving that are separate from criminal investigations. |
| Corrective steps | Not required. Painful punishment is the only way to establish deterrence and law obedience. | One way to deal with crime is that the aggressive person(s) make(s) corrective steps towards the victims or the community, e.g. by fixing the damage or by apologising in writing. |
| Reconciliation gestures | Police officers are not required to make any positive gestures toward civilians in general, or Arab civilians in particular. It is not in police interests to develop long-term relationships that are based on trust and working on behalf of civilians. | One of the main principles of building a connecting authority is the police's ability to extend positive gestures to the communities in which they work, which demonstrate flexible thinking and acting without compromising the safety of either civilians and their property or of the police force. |
| (Omer, 2011; Gilad, 2013) | | |

 

# Examples of police activity using the principles of connecting authority

## Example of presence and closeness

I serve as a consultant for establishing trust and co-operation between police and the Arab community in the town of Tamra in northern Israel, home to some 30,000 people, most of them Muslims. Prior to building a local police station a few months before the project started, the people that lived in the town characterised the police's presence as either insufficient – 'a lack of policing' – or excessive – 'over-policing'. What this meant was that there was generally a minimal police presence, which increased the anger and alienation of the civilians, but that when police intervention was needed it was heavy handed, resulting in increased anger and resentment among the residents.

As part of the responsibilities of the police's Department for Service Accessibility for Arab Society, organisational consultants started working in several Arab towns and villages in an effort to change the relationship between police and local communities. The process in Tamra began by establishing a local steering committee, consisting of the mayor and municipal department heads, respected religious/community leaders, educators and the local police commanders.

This steering committee met for a series of six sessions, which were designed to promote closeness, familiarity and trust among participants. During these sessions, civilians and police officers described their expectations of each other, expressed constructive criticism and identified mutual goals. At first, the two sides tended to blame each other for the way things are. However, the group facilitators urged participants to adopt an open, non-judgemental attitude and listen carefully to what the others had to say.

By the end of the process, basic trust and willingness to co-operate had developed. The guiding principle was to co-operate in order to create an environment of confidence and safety for the residents of Tamra. Setting this shared goal allowed for both sides to overcome the obstacles and emotional baggage that stood between the two parties. Both sides committed themselves to find the best way to a better future.

In one of the sessions, a local attorney expressed his amazement by saying, 'For us to sit together with the police and discuss problems in our town with no aggressive interaction – that's strange'. The station commander replied, 'The police have concluded that we need to change our attitude and be more attentive and accessible'. The commander thus demonstrated that he was not afraid to admit that the police needed to change its ways in dealing with the Arab population, and this admission did not reduce his sense of self-respect or lower his self-confidence.

## Examples of co-operation

### Educational initiative: *Paving a Way*

As an organisational consultant in Tamra, my role was made up of a few components:

1. Helping police commanders and civilians to create relationships of trust through direct encounters, where I facilitated discussions and highlighted everyone's ability to contain criticism and stick to agreed goals.
2. Using the connecting authority approach to help collaboration between police and civilians. My responsibility was to encourage and help convey information, shaping a united perception among partners, increasing presence and persistence when carrying out non-violent and determined actions to decrease crime. It was also to emphasise and establish trust-building steps, corrective steps and gestures of good will on the part of the police.

For example, a programme was designed in which police officers gave lectures and performed experiential activities with teenagers in one of the local schools. The programme was prepared in several sessions with the school principal, educational consultants and the PTA chairperson. This sent a message of co-operation and defused the opposition to police activity within the school that some parents felt. The programme included simulations of real events, with policemen role-playing teens and vice versa, followed by discussions about police duties and the teens' negative attitudes in response. Another activity involved a meeting with the student council, where police officers asked members for advice regarding police activity and what they would be willing to do to minimise crime in their town. After one of the lectures, one student said to the station commander, 'Thank you for coming and showing us that police officers are also people!'

In another example, in Tamra, a committee was established to deal with conflicts between large extended families. It included municipal officials, religious and other leaders who are respected by both local families and police officers. My job was to help all participants to develop an integrated model for these conflict resolution situations, which were completely different from classic policing. Together we produced the following model:

 

1. The police arrive, assess the situation and decide whether to detain the involved parties at the station for questioning.
2. Assuming there is no evidence requiring legal procedures, an intervention team is called, including the mayor, deputy mayor, and others who are acceptable to both sides of the conflict. A traditional routine in Arab society is calling together a 'reconciliation committee' of respected community figures who mediate in cases of conflicts between families. However, over time, this mechanism has lost its power due to the weakening status of respected figures in the community and the younger generation's tendency to ignore their decisions. In this model, police involvement reinforces and re-validates these old routines, provided that both sides agree to the observance of state law as a fundamental and crucial condition to continue the team's work.
3. The team advises the two sides to reach an agreement to end the conflict, which they must sign and promise to keep. The intervention team continues to follow up and make sure that the agreement is carried out and peace is maintained, using the three-contact approach described below.
4. In cases where there has been a minor felony (i.e. threats, swearing or pushing, with no physical damage), the team suggests to the involved parties that instead of facing a judge and risking a criminal record, they may report to a police prosecutor who would order corrective steps. The head of the police prosecutors in this unit was also introduced to the connecting authority and agreed to follow the approved procedure. This option in the model has many advantages:
   a. it is presented as a gesture of good will on the part of the police
   b. no criminal records are opened
   c. the prosecutor may, as a last resort, order corrective steps instead of classic punishment, such as writing a letter of apology or fixing damage to property.

   This way, positive communication is created between the disputed families, diminishing attitudes of aggression and revenge.

# Conclusion

The advantage of the connecting authority model is that it is not limited to teaching behavioural principles to single police officers. The model enables the entire police force and society to develop comprehensive strategies for powerful non-violent actions, conveying the message that determined efforts are being made to prevent crime, particularly violence, in a way that minimises physical and emotional harm to civilians and leaves room for an open dialogue between the police and civilians.

Developing such a strategy is extremely important for establishing trust among the Arab population in Israel. The connecting authority model uses public media to advertise their determination to fight crime while minimising unnecessary harm to individuals or groups. Through connecting authority, the individual policeman and the police as a whole can implant in civilians a sense that there is an alternative means of conflict resolution and an effective way forward that does not rely on violence or on 'ruler/ruled' or 'winner/loser' relationships.

This approach contains the potential for change, from the dynamics of hatred and fear to those of trust and partnership. If the police would agree to take on the principles of connecting authority, this could lead to informed and planned structuring of conflicts and could prevent conflict situations from deteriorating into uncontrollable confrontations, both emotionally and physically.

As demonstrated in Tamra, this can be achieved by creating partnerships between community leaders and local officials, introducing 'support networks' to law enforcement, along with the ability to actively seek constructive means with which to negotiate and reach agreements with the minority community.

The principle of transparency and publicity requires the police to develop a public relations strategy to distribute constructive messages before, during and after confrontations with individuals and social groups. The principles of persistence, de-escalation and support free police officers from desperate attempts to reach an immediate resolution and deal with each and every occurrence of defiance. This new stance is not to be perceived as weakness, but as authority that builds its strength on continual, consistent, determined and planned processes.

Thus, the connecting authority approach presents an inspiring framework with a great variety of planned, non-violent action, persistence and tolerant resistance. Self-control and pride in the police's professional identity can be maintained, strengthened and given a complete new meaning when police officers are taught non-violent methods. This non-violent resistance approach therefore represents the chance for a joint, safe and effective partnership response to crime. At the same time, it represents a person and service-oriented perspective in problem-solving, that is based on respecting others and their weaknesses and limitations. This allows both sides to develop different perspectives of each other and to move beyond hatred, aggression, negative perceptions and stereotypes, thereby enabling more constructive communication and relationships.

## References

Ali N (2014) Violence and crime in Israeli-Arab society: a governmental conspiracy or cultural crime? (in Hebrew). Haifa: University of Haifa.

Bar-Tal D (2007). Sociopsychological foundations of intractable conflicts. *American Behavioral Scientist* **50** (11) 1430–1453.

Bom H & Wiebenga E (2017) Connecting Authority, towards a new authority based on nonviolent resistance (in Dutch). *Journal of Psychotherapy* **43** (4) 269–289

Carmeli A & Shamir N (2000) Police violence towards citizens (in Hebrew). *Ministry of Internal Security.* Chief Scientist's Office.

Gilad Z (2013) Modifying the constructive struggle approach to police work in Israel (in Hebrew). Tel Aviv University: Ph.D. dissertation.

Gimshi D (2003) Police in a democracy (in Hebrew). Jerusalem: Police Department of Israel.

Gofer A & Ben porat G (2013) Policing a divided society Pardes.

Harpaz A (2008) Community policing and police officers' attitudes toward minority groups in Israel: contact with minority communities and changing prejudices (in Hebrew). Haifa: University of Haifa.

Hasisi B (2005) Policing and citizenship in a torn society: police-minority relationships in Israel (in Hebrew). PhD dissertation. Haifa: University of Haifa.

Hasisi B (2014) Attitude survey: Partnership and cooperation in the relationships between Israel Police and Israeli-Arab society (in Hebrew). An initiative of the Abraham Foundation.

Hasisi B (2016) Police, Politics, and Culture in a Deeply Divided Society. In: Zamir, Weisburd and Hasisi (Eds.) *Policing in Israel Studying Crime Control, Community Policing, and Counterterrorism* (pp87–107). Boca Raton: CRC Press.

Omer H (2011) The New Authority: Family, school, community. London and New York: Cambridge University Press.

Reuss–Ianni E (1983) Two Cultures of Policing: Street cops and management cops. New Jersey: Transaction Books.

Samocha S (2000) *An ethnic democracy: Israel as a prototype*. In: Gavison & Hacker (Eds). The Jewish-Arab Rift in Israel: A reader (pp277–307) (in Hebrew). Jerusalem: The Israel Democracy Institute.

Samocha S (2005) Arab-Jewish Relationship Index (in Hebrew). Haifa: the Jewish-Arab Center, University of Haifa.

Santo Y & Ali N (2008) Policing in the Israeli-Arab Society: A survey among Israeli-Arab citizens (in Hebrew). Israel: The Ministry of the Interior.

Skolnick JH (1993) Justice without trial. In: Weisburd & Uchida (Eds). *Police Innovation and Control of the Police* (pp13–31). Springer-Verlag, New York, 1993.

VaanMaanen (1978) On watching the watchers. In: Manning & Van Maanen (Eds) *Policing: A view from the street* (pp221–237). Goodyear.

# Chapter 9: NVR in a youth justice context

**By Zoe McLeod and Gill Westwood**

## Introduction

This chapter looks at the application of non-violent resistance parenting principles to the context of a Youth Offending Service (YOS). It is interesting to note that many of the principles of non-violent resistance – de-escalation, acts of resistance, reconciliation gestures, self-care and the announcement – find parallels in the YOS's work to support young people to change.

The chapter starts with an overview of a London borough and its YOS. This is followed by comparing relevant theories that are currently used in youth offending contexts with key NVR principles, which we highlight with examples from our practice. We will finally draw out some learning points from our experience.

The term 'family' can encompass many relationships, including but not limited to parents, grandparents, older siblings, looked-after young people and foster families, and we have been privileged to work with many families each with their own unique identities and structures. For the purposes of clarity in this chapter, we will use terms such as 'parent', 'parents' and 'carer' interchangeably, but we wish to acknowledge the richness and uniqueness of every family.

## Context

Our YOS is situated in a culturally diverse London borough which is the vibrant home to over 270,000 people. One in five of its residents is under 18 years old, making it one of the youngest boroughs in the metropolitan area. It also suffers from some of the highest child poverty rates in the UK, with high costs of housing and domestic overcrowding (Lewisham.gov.uk, 2018). It is one of the fastest developing and greenest parts of south-east London with over a fifth of the borough made up of parkland and open spaces. Within this context, 0.7% of young people aged between 10 and 18 will at some point come to the attention of the Borough Youth Offending Services (Lewishamjsna, 2018).

Youth Offending Services were established in England and Wales by the Crime and Disorder Act (1998) and consist of multi-disciplinary teams overseen by local government. YOS teams have the responsibility to facilitate the sentences passed down by youth courts and to consider the balance of care and control in their work. Young people commit criminal acts in the context of their developmental needs, environmental influences, educational experience and level of welfare. Within this framework YOS practitioners are required to consider parenting as both an influence and a resource when working with young people in trouble.

Perceptions of parental deficiency have long been regarded as a causal factor in anti-social behaviour and offending (Pearson, 1994) and the Crime and Disorder Act (1998) gave courts the power to consider issuing a 'Parenting Order' to any parent of an offending young person. These Parenting Orders were designed to ensure a carer's engagement in correcting and guiding young people who have contravened the law.

Local councils determine what strategies are employed to engage families and support them to manage their child's offending behaviour. The intention of this borough is that work with parents should be collaborative rather than coercive. Rather than use Parenting Orders, the YOS shows its recognition of the importance of family by employing a parenting officer who is a systemic family therapist, as well as a team of three functional family therapists. The wider YOS team has been familiarised with systemic approaches and our particular YOS has an embedded team of Child and Adolescent Mental Health Service (CAMHS) workers. These CAMHS workers offer support to young people with mental health needs and their families.

The parenting officer works with carers in a variety of ways including helping them navigate the youth justice system, aiding them with practical matters such as housing, employment and education, and offering them support for family relationships. The Functional Family Therapy team work with cases where the young person elects to join their parent to engage in family work.

YOS family work is multi-disciplinary and systemic; NVR shares this systemic underpinning and so fits well into our context. Interventions are carefully sequenced so that families are not overwhelmed by multiple agencies offering involvement at the same time. Transitions and endings are planned with families.

## Target group

The YOS works with young people aged ten to 17 who have come to the attention of the police and courts. Many children in the youth justice system are known to come from the poorest and most disadvantaged families and communities, and many of them face multiple other challenges. Speech, language or communication difficulties are estimated to stand at 60%, and approximately one in four young offenders has a diagnosed learning need. One-third of young people in custody have an identified mental health condition, which is three times higher than that of the general population. UK studies have indicated an ADHD rate of 43% in 14-year-old youths in custody, which significantly exceeds the adolescent community prevalence rate of 5%. Research also tells us that young people from Black, Asian and Minority Ethnic (BAME) backgrounds are more likely to be stopped, searched, arrested, charged and more stringently sentenced than their white peers, meaning that families attending the YOS are disproportionately drawn from these communities (Sloane & Allison, 2015).

The young people presenting at the YOS are considered more likely to self-medicate with alcohol or drugs and may have been exposed to a higher number of adverse childhood experiences (ACE) (Smith & Thornberry, 1995) such as domestic abuse, homelessness, bereavement, family separation and long periods alone.

## The relevance of NVR

The intersection of experiences of racism, socio-economic disadvantage, poor mental health, learning needs and ACE can render both parent and child more vulnerable to a range of adverse experiences including anxiety and reduced emotional self-regulation. Adolescent to parent violence and abuse (APVA) may be one expression of this, and NVR is a particularly appropriate intervention for these families.

APVA in a youth justice context may manifest in formal charges such as criminal damage in the home, or as an offence against the person charge such as common assault or actual bodily harm to a family member. The Home Office's *Information Guide: Adolescent to parent violence and abuse (APVA)* (2015) highlights that many parents experiencing violence at home are reluctant to report incidents to the police due to fears of removal and/or criminalisation of the child. This leaves parents in the unenviable position of being victims of the aggression, informants of the offence as well as advocates for the perpetrator.

Parents of young people under 17 are expected to attend the police station, court hearings and YOS meetings with their child and they are aware of dominant social discourses suggesting that poor parenting may cause youth transgression. Parents who are victims of their child's offending thus feel additionally punished and helpless.

Parents report feeling that they are isolated and silenced within their families, communities and workplaces, and they disclose to us that entry into the youth justice system is the first time they have been offered help with their young person. Some carers also express a sense of disappointment that their child has had to offend in order for the relevant support to be made available. Parents of young people convicted of unrelated offences may also use this contact as an opportunity to enlist help and disclose their experience of APVA. Experiences of APVA have been associated with family breakdown and youth homelessness; these are additional risk factors which increase the chances of a young person re-offending. This means that supporting carers with NVR parenting directly addresses some of the concerns of the youth justice system.

Most programmes offered to parents of offenders have been developed as preventative approaches and are generally designed to meet the needs of younger children. NVR acknowledges that parents may not be in a position to impose their authority or enforce rewards and punishments. Parents in NVR are therefore supported to create a secure climate in which to address the violence within their families, which addresses the need to keep themselves and other family members safe. An NVR group provides a contained space for parents to share their experiences of parenting children with violent, aggressive or controlling behaviours, without fear of being blamed or shamed. They can draw strength, not only from the course strategies offered, but from the group as a whole. Parents become increasingly supportive of each other as the group progresses. NVR's focus on sibling experience can help address parents' concerns about the direct and indirect impact of the behaviour of the index child on their other children. Evidence indicates a higher incidence of offending among siblings of young people with a criminal history (Beijers *et al*, 2017).

## Theory and literature

A number of theories and models currently inform the practice of YOS interventions with young people. It is interesting to note that NVR complements the principles of each of these models in different ways.

**Desistance theories** focus on young people's development of a future-orientated pro-social self-identity (Maruna & LeBel, 2012). Young people are encouraged to take control of the present and to expand and explore their understanding of themselves and others to build a more hopeful view of their future (Gray, 2013). Desistance theory promotes 'valuing people for who they are and for what they could become, rather than judging, rejecting or containing them for what they have done' (McNeill *et al*, 2012).

 

NVR invites parents to resume or take on their vital role in transforming the young person's view of themselves. It provides tools to repair ruptured relationships and to challenge and renew family expectations as carers resist escalation and submission.

**The Good Lives Model** is used in National Probation Service practice and adapted for use with younger people. It considers the function of behaviours in meeting young people's needs. The model recognises these needs as 'primary goods'. 'Goods' include relatedness, community and inner peace. Some young people attempt to meet these needs through behaviours such as controlling or coercive interpersonal relationships, gang involvement and drug use or self-harm (Ward & Fortune, 2013). The Good Lives Model encourages young people to meet these needs in other ways.

NVR complements this by supporting parents to recognise and meet their child's needs in more collaborative and relationship-enhancing ways.

**Trauma-informed approaches** have increasingly influenced practice models in youth justice; 86% of young people in the Youth Justice System may have experienced trauma (Skuse & Matthew, 2015). The focus of trauma-informed work includes building trusting relationships, hearing the voice of the young person and recognising fight, flight and freeze responses. YOS practitioners seek to provide a working environment which reduces stress and anxiety and acknowledges the importance of families managing these environments.

NVR's use of de-escalation to reduce the threat of violence and aggression can help families to regulate difficult emotions and avoid becoming emotionally accelerated. NVR's emphasis on creating safety and rebuilding trust and security can assist families in the development of alternative means of communication through acts of reconciliation and resistance, as well as parental presence.

**Attachment Theory** tells us that young people in adolescence need to individuate their own identity and to master responsibility for their independence. These activities are difficult to accomplish and can be painful for parents who must prepare, permit, and accept these changes. When young people transgress, parent's trust is deeply harmed, and when that disobedience manifests in violence or intimidation at home, the wounds are uniquely painful. Controlling and coercive behaviours frustrate the growth of new relational patterns.

Much of the research available to guide criminal justice work has been developed with adult populations and the maturation of young people is a vital consideration in their application.

Non-violent resistance can provide a framework for parents to acknowledge developmental needs, rebuild trust and create new capacity in their relationships.

**Restorative Justice Practices** are increasingly being embedded in youth justice. The independent evaluation commissioned by the Ministry of Justice identified that involvement in a restorative process reduced re-offending rates by 14% (Restorative Justice in youth offending teams, 2015). Young people attending the YOS may have a history of ruptured relationships and ambiguous endings in different areas of their lives. However, good restorative work recognises that young people cannot be expected to empathise with their victims until their needs for security are sufficiently met (Carroll, 2017).

NVR's focus on repairing relationships, reconciliation and improved communication enables young people and their families to begin to engage in more formal restorative work.

**The Contextual Safeguarding Framework** (Firmin, 2018) recognises that young people are at risk of sexual and criminal exploitation by their peers in community spaces. The model broadens the scope of safeguarding beyond family and individual interventions to the community and wider environment. Emerging trends in youth offending suggest that those who criminally exploit young people are increasingly innovative in securing young people's obedience and silence through means of direct abuse, threats, shame, debt and coercion. They actively isolate young people at a time when parental and adult guidance are most needed.

The invitation for adults to enter young people's physical domains, such as parks and playgrounds, will be familiar to parents who participate in NVR. Extending parental and adult presence into these spaces, through organised networks, is a tool to protect children who may be vulnerable to.

The parental presence of NVR does not rely on coercion to engage the child. Instead, parents are supported to reconnect by acknowledging their own hurt and changing the patterns of submission and dominance that can contribute to the child's self-destructive behaviours. Research suggests that peers rather than family are the dominant influence in creating social norms for young people in the UK and US (Brechwald & Prinstein, 2011). NVR can create a safe place within the family for young people who are experiencing danger, pressure and uncertainty. This can enable them to better question the social norms they may be experiencing in their peer group.

 

## Description of the practice

Given the shame and blame discourses they experience, it is no surprise that parents are cautious about attending group programmes. YOS practitioners are familiar with the structure and purpose of NVR and are skilled at recognising when it will be useful and referring parents to the programme. Approaches to potential parents are warm, creative, persistent and sensitive. Parents are offered individual sessions that preview and teach the NVR material and can give some familiarity and understanding before they are introduced to other group members. The relationship that develops with facilitators over this time can be a factor in encouraging the parents to attend.

Some carers attend NVR after completing a Functional Family Therapy intervention. Parents might initially attend alone, or with other family members or supporters. Where young people are co-parented, both parents are encouraged to attend together or separately depending on their wishes and availability. Parents may be working with other professionals and these workers are also invited to participate in the sessions. A family support worker who has attended the session is able to support the family's progress more effectively and to build on the work during the week, ideally ensuring that any strategies they offer do not conflict with the principles of NVR.

NVR groups at the YOS are small; we have found that a group of between four and eight members works well. Parents are given a timetable of potential session times and dates and select their availability. This is collated to inform the scheduling of the next course. This simple choice can be empowering for some parents, demonstrating an authentic interest in their needs, with the result that they may feel more encouraged to attend. Parents are offered an initial taster session and the courses run for between ten and 12 weeks. Groups are facilitated by two NVR trained co-facilitators and, where possible, an additional facilitator from CAMHS.

The small size of the YOS cohort means that young people are potentially socially connected by school community and sometimes criminal association. Risk planning before group sessions with parents has therefore been essential. Discussions about confidentiality allow parents to make informed choices about joining the group: some parents choose not to refer to their child by name or school to preserve anonymity, and carers may ask to only be contacted via work email, or may choose to prepare a response in case their child questions where they are going. Parents are reminded that confidentiality is a shared responsibility which is in place to ensure the safety of everyone, and simple oversights could put families and young people in danger. Parent's concerns are carefully considered.

## Lived experience practitioners

We have been privileged to work with graduate parents from the NHS trust that first developed this group programme, but it has been a challenge for us to grow our own pool of 'graduate', or 'lived experience' practitioners. We recognise that graduate parents are a huge strength of NVR. However, we have to balance this with the fact that it may be difficult for YOS parents to step into this role. For NVR-trained parents, patterns and challenges of progress and setback will be familiar; for parents in the criminal justice system, the impact of their child relapsing or re-offending in the community can be devastating and far-reaching. Lived experience practitioners are generous and sensitive in sharing their unique insights and knowledge with other families, and it has been our concern that this may be an unfair expectation for parents whose parenting has been brought under public scrutiny. The role of the YOS in a young person's life is also time bound, making it less likely that parents will want to continue engagement with our service beyond the duration of their child's Court Order. The small size of the YOS community also makes it more difficult to manage issues around confidentiality and safety.

# Practice examples

Families attending NVR are often living in highly stressful environments and have been managing unstable and risky situations over long periods without respite. Providing a calm space where parents can feel valued, respected, heard and cared for is a priority in planning this work. Simple considerations like providing a comfortable private room and home-baked cake, fruit, refreshments and tissues can make an enormous difference. Parents who report that they are constantly responding to unpredictable behaviours often benefit from a safe and predictable environment which can give them the space to find their voice. The intimate size of the groups enables the development of close supportive relationships between parents, which allows them to be authentic and vulnerable, and to express their emotions freely.

### Practice example 1: Hannah

*Hannah had previously expressed her reluctance to join an NVR group. She was worried about talking to new people and discussing her son's offending in front of parents who might know his reputation. We were able to meet with Hannah before the group and talk her through the plan that had been designed for the introductory session. We described the times when she might be asked to speak and reassured her that she could remain quiet if she chose. We helped Hannah prepare answers she would be comfortable giving to other parents should they question her directly. We were also able to negotiate our role in supporting Hannah to make use of the session.*

 

## Practice example 2: Sarah

*Sarah reported that she could not attend NVR as her daughter, Ann, had refused to babysit Sarah's youngest child. This was in protest that her mother was intending to attend the group and invest more time in her elder brother who had caused so much damage to their home. We met the mother and daughter at their home and were able to discuss the overall plan of NVR and recruit Ann's vital help. Ann became an energetic support to her mother and was able to rebuild her relationship with her brother, as well as identify her own need for support.*

## Practice example 3: facilitator's commitment announcement

Throughout our work with parents, we, as practitioners, have sought opportunities to personify the principles of NVR. In sessions, we offer our ground rules in the form of an announcement.

*We, Gill, Zoe and ....... are dedicated to offering parents the best help we can. As the facilitators of this course we want you to know that your physical and emotional safety are important to us.*

*We will do everything we can to ensure that this feels like a safe place where you can talk as much or as little as you want.*

*We will not talk about our discussions in this room elsewhere, unless we have serious concerns about physical or emotional harm to yourself or another.*

*We will also do everything we can to ensure that you do not feel alone in your situation.*

## Practice example 4: ending a course

We send a card to parents at the end of the course written in the language of an announcement, stating that we support carers in the changes they are trying to make and acknowledging all they are doing to make those changes.

*Dear Helen,*

*We wanted to say thank you for being such a valuable part of this group and for your warmth and humour. Thank you for your courage to share your challenges and successes; this has been inspiring for us all. You have really helped to energise us with your willingness to try something new and to take a chance.*

*We wanted to let you know that we fully support you as you continue to practice de-escalation and as you continue to build relationships with small acts of kindness to your boys. We will always remember your amazing positivity as you manage such a full-on household and remember you as a mum who keeps on going even when the going is tough*

*With our very best wishes*

### Practice example 5: other tips

- Any concerns among the group about potential escalation of tension or conflict gives an opportunity to explore and apply the ideas of de-escalation in a safe environment.
- Lecturing and long explanations can be experienced as patronising at best and escalation at worst, and it is important that facilitators are alert to their own tendency to be too 'wordy' and to monitor themselves.
- As facilitators, we model reconciliation gestures and acts of resistance. Each session is viewed as an experience of self-care and we always end with a relaxation exercise.
- In order to develop good practice, it has been valuable to make use of debriefing periods following sessions, as well as setting aside practice days to review the application and success of the groups.
- Meeting with other NVR practitioners has encouraged further development, fidelity to the ethos of the model and provided the energy of peer support.

## Learning points

Increasingly, when beginning a course we are explicit from the outset that parents need to be ready to try something very different and that they will be challenged to examine some of their core beliefs about parenting. As we have become more practised in running NVR courses, and have experience of working with parents who have attended NVR with other providers, we have become conscious of aspects of our teaching that are open to misinterpretation. A misunderstanding some parents struggle with is that NVR is solely about de-escalating and that this means avoiding all conflict with the young person and submitting to their demands to avoid future conflict. It is therefore critical that sufficient weight is given to the importance of acts of resistance and parental presence. We are consciously reviewing ways to build more focus on these elements into our course.

We try to make our language accessible in all our courses. For example, we refer to Reconciliation Gestures as 'acts of kindness'. We have also devised and used visual supports for some of the concepts of NVR, which are tailored to fit with individual group experiences.

Some parents are offered a range of different interventions at the same time or in quick succession. The focus and direction of these interventions can be very different and sometimes conflicting. Parents are sometimes left paralysed by professionals instructing them to implement a range of contradictory strategies.

 

We are working towards adopting a Team around the Worker (Adolescent Mentalisation-Based Integrative Therapy (AMBIT)) approach to this dilemma: a lead professional selected by the family co-ordinates interventions with professionals to ensure a coherent proposal of intervention (Bevington *et al*, 2013). If this approach is not successful we may reluctantly withdraw the offer of NVR while other statutory agencies complete their work so as not to contribute to parental confusion.

Gathering valid evidence from parents about the efficacy of NVR is an ongoing challenge. We recognise the need for both quantitative and qualitative evaluation and we have used the SCORE 15 and SUDS tools as well as a final narrative questionnaire. This process is always under review.

In our experience, it is not enough simply to adopt NVR as a parenting strategy into a YOS. We believe that it is the responsibility of the workers to remain curious and committed to adapting their approaches, including NVR, to fit the parents we work with. We have given some examples of potential barriers to attendance and demonstrated how we have extended the NVR announcement by delivering joint facilitator announcements at the beginning and end of the group programme with parents, thereby making the NVR approach more tailored to the specific needs of the YOS context.

## References

Beijers J, Bijleveld C, van de Weijer S & Liefbroer A (2017) "All in the family?" The relationship between sibling offending and offending risk. *Journal of Developmental and Life-Course Criminology* **3** (1) pp1–14.

Bevington D, Fuggle P, Fonagy P, Target M & Asen E (2013) Innovations in practice: Adolescent Mentalization-Based Integrative Therapy (AMBIT)–a new integrated approach to working with the most hard to reach adolescents with severe complex mental health needs. *Child and Adolescent Mental Health* **18** (1) pp46–51.

Brechwald WA & Prinstein MJ (2011) Beyond homophily: a decade of advances in understanding peer influence processes. *Journal of Research on Adolescence* **21** (1) pp166–179.

Carroll JC (2017) *Restorative Justice Training* [online].

Restorative Justice Council (2015) *Restorative Justice in Youth Offending Teams – Information pack* [online]. Available at: https://restorativejustice.org.uk/sites/default/files/resources/files/kn1b_info_packs%20(2)%20yot_0.pdf (accessed November 2018).

Firmin C (2018) Contextual risk, individualised responses: an assessment of safeguarding responses to nine cases of peer-on-peer abuse. *Child abuse review* **27** (1) pp42–57.

Gray P (2013) *Report of Research on Youth Offending Team Partnerships and the Social Context of Youth Crime* [online]. Plymouth: Plymouth University. Available at: https://pearl.plymouth.ac.uk/handle/10026.1/9007 (accessed November 2018).

Home Office (2015) *Information Guide: Adolescent to Parent Violence and Abuse* [online]. Available at: https://assets.publishing.service.gov.uk/government/uploads/system/uploads/attachment_data/file/732573/APVA.pdf (accessed November 2018).

 

Lewisham.gov.uk (2018) 2011 *Census Second Release* [online]. Available at: http://www.lewisham.gov.uk/inmyarea/Documents/2011CensusSecondReleaseDec2012.pdf (accessed November 2018).

Lewishamjsna.org.uk (2018). *Lewisham's Joint Strategic Needs Assessment (JSNA)* [online]. Available at: www.lewishamjsna.org.uk/lewishams-joint-strategic-needs-assessment-jsna (accessed November 2018).

Maruna S & LeBel TP (2012) The desistance paradigm in correctional practice: from programmes to lives. In: F McNeill, P Raynor and C Trotter (Eds) *Offender Supervision* (pp91–114). Willan.

McNeill F, Farrall S, Lightowler C & Maruna S (2012) *How and Why People Stop Offending: Discovering desistance*. Institute for Research and Innovation in Social Services.

Pearson G (1994) 'Youth, crime and society'. In: M Maguire, R Morgan and R Reiner (Eds.) *The Oxford Handbook of Criminology*. Oxford: Clarendon Press.

Skuse T & Matthew J (2015) The Trauma Recovery Model: Sequencing youth justice interventions for young people with complex needs. *Prison Service Journal* **220** pp16–24.

Smith C & Thornberry TP (1995) The relationship between childhood maltreatment and adolescent involvement in delinquency. *Criminology* **33** (4) pp451–481.

Sloane A & Allison E (2015) Sharp rise in the proportion of young black and ethnic minority prisoners. *The Guardian* **11 March**.

Ward T & Fortune C (2013) The Good Lives Model: aligning risk reduction with promoting offenders' personal goals. *European Journal of Probation* **5** (2) 29–46.

 

# Chapter 10: Reflections on NVR specialist groups for parents whose children are affected by gangs and child sexual exploitation

**By Elisabeth Heismann, Julie Pierzchniak and Jane Prescott**

## Introduction

There is hardly anyone who has not come across headlines such as the following five:

- '*The government must get to grips with youth violence and gangs*' (Umunna, 2016), '*Gang members "filming rape attacks on schoolgirls as young as 13 in south Birmingham"*' (Oldham, 2017).
- '*Knife crime up 14% because gang warfare is becoming "embedded in our culture"*' (Walker, 2017).
- '*British youth are "the most unpleasant and violent in the world": Damning verdict of writer as globe reacts to riots*' (Moran & Hall, 2011).
- '*Youth crime soars in last five years as gang culture takes grip*' (Clark, 2008).
- '*Parents need more help to protect their children from gangs*' (Firmin, 2012).

Gangs and child sexual exploitation (CSE) are closely connected to drugs and crime in many London boroughs and some other areas of the UK. The south London borough in which we provide a specialist group was the 19th most deprived out of 326 local authorities in the UK in 2010 (Hines 2012). Of the working age residents in the borough, 4.8% were claiming job seekers allowance[4], of which 12% were in the age group below 24 and of which 37% had been claiming for more than six months (Hines, 2012). Considering these demographics, the attractiveness of gangs to young people, particularly organised crime operating as a business, is not surprising. The borough was ranked fourth highest out of 32 London boroughs for assault and third highest for injury offences. The Safer Communities *Strategy for Tackling Serious Youth Violence* report (unpublished) stated that youth crime accounted for 49.2% of crimes where the age of the perpetrator was known.

Of the three authors of this chapter, two practitioners have been involved in generic NVR group programmes (Day & Heismann, 2010) in this borough for more than 10 years. The third author works as a deputy head in a school for boys with social emotional and mental health (SEMH) difficulties in another borough but wanted to learn about the specialist NVR group programme and used the placement as facilitator as part of her facilitator training.

In this chapter we will describe an NVR group programme with a specialist focus on gangs and CSE that took place over nine months in a London borough. We will describe the uniqueness of this journey through the authors' own experiences as facilitators, the experiences of graduate parents involved in the processes and our learning, findings and reflections. Finally, we will discuss our vision that NVR is a shared practice with a common language that can be used widely to build safe and connected communities.

## The need to develop a specialist NVR group programme

Based on our experience of parents who are known to agencies but who do not meet the criteria to access CAMHS, we came to the conclusion that the generic NVR programme in CAMHS did not meet the additional needs of parents whose children are involved in or affected by gangs or by CSE. Some of the graduate parents from the generic NVR programmes who had children with gang involvement and CSE became involved as co-facilitators in our specialist groups.

Our objectives for the specialist groups were to support parents to accept the risks posed by gangs and CSE, to take a non-violent and committed stand against

4 The London average is 4% and the national rate 3.8% (Hines, 2012).

 

violence and abuse, to de-escalate conflicts and re-build family relationships, to increase vigilant care and parental presence and to break the cycle of silence, isolation, shame and guilt. We therefore designed the specialist groups based on the generic programme but we altered it in the following ways:

- We made it a longer programme: 14 weeks instead of 12.
- We included individual home visits for four weeks before the group started. The purpose of the four visits was to meet with the referrer and the family to establish their goals, to start building a relationship of trust with them and to introduce them to some of the NVR concepts. These visits were extremely valuable as some parents were unable to attend the group afterwards but expressed to us and their referrers that they had found the support from the home visits very helpful. '*I so wish I had been able to attend,*' said one such parent, '*this should be available to all parents who are struggling.*' An additional benefit of the home visits for us all was that we managed to see other family members, including the young people concerned, and often recruited their support for the programme. We also distributed some material and information about NVR, thereby planting a seed for possible future attendance.
- We created a steering group with stake holders of gangs and CSE experts (e.g. the gangs link worker for the borough and the chair of the borough's CSE panel), which met four times during the group: they helped us with presentations and presenters. There was a sense of mutual accountability in which information from the group could inform new ways of working and incorporate innovative perspectives into their own agencies.
- We incorporated presentations from local agencies (outlined in *Graduate parent involvement*, below): presenters from various key organisations made themselves available for half an hour at the beginning of a group evening.
- We gave additional support to group members, including phone calls, home visits and attendance at safeguarding conferences.
- We developed our own vision of NVR as a shared practice with a common language that can be used in specialist contexts to build safer and more connected communities.

The findings and learning points in this chapter are particularly drawn from the last group we ran, which combined parents whose children were affected by gangs and by CSE, but we also include our more general learning from the last five years and how we applied it to this particular group and context.

## Graduate parent involvement

As in all generic NVR group work, the participation of graduate parents was key in this group. We included four graduate parents in the specialist group, which allowed us to have two in each sub-group. This inclusivity was an essential component of the programme and is also described as a main feature in the Just Therapy service in New Zealand (Waldegrave, *et al*, 2003). Parents could talk from their own experiences of having their sons in gangs or their daughters groomed and sexually exploited.

One graduate parent said, '*As a graduate parent facilitator I really enjoyed sharing my own experiences with the parents and showing them that it is ok to let the barriers down and break the silence*'. Another commented, '*Although I was a fairly inexperienced member of the team, I was greatly valued, and my opinion was appreciated... The parents were able to identify with the graduate parent on an emotional level*'.

Graduate parents participated in a training programme about gangs organised by the borough's safer community team, which all facilitators attended before the programme started. They then came along to the home visits where they often encouraged new participants, particularly those who were reluctant or did not think that they or their children had a problem. One graduate parent was surprised by the differences between the participants of the generic groups she had co-facilitated before and the prospective participants in this specialist group:

> *'I was struck by how different the parents seemed to the parents of the CAMHS NVR course. A 'typical parent' on the generic course seems broken, at the end of their tether, unable to cope and afraid to ask for help. The parents we encountered on the home visits tended to be very strong, protective and defensive of their children. They tended to be secretive, distrusting of professionals, not afraid to say what they think.'*

During the home visits, we often met the young people who were originally referred to us and were able to see them and their 'harmful' behaviour in a new light. As one graduate parent said:

> *'The visits gave a human element to the 'gang' members' who had been discussed in terms of offending behaviour. We were fortunate to meet some of the young people, which was interesting. It gave us an insight into how their parents viewed their young people. Some of them were an absolute pleasure to meet which gave us an understanding of how some parents could be unaware*

*of the gravity of the situations their young people were finding themselves in as the children were hiding their 'street' behaviour from the family.'*

This enabled the graduate parents to edit their own testimonies by also highlighting the positive sides of their own children and how they were initially reluctant to face up to the grim reality of their own children's behaviour outside the home and how the NVR group and the presentations enabled them to face up to it.

During the group programme, new participants sometimes formed their closest bonds with one particular graduate parent, often those who had accompanied us to the initial home visits. They would sit next to their 'favourite' graduate parent or try to grab them for a brief conversation before or after the group, or during the breaks.

Although some new participants shared their weekly news with their favourite graduate parent on a one-to-one basis, it was made clear to all participants at the beginning of the program that all facilitators would discuss any additional information about them and their children in the post-sessions. During the professional presentations, for example in relation to missing children, drugs and the experience of young people with the social justice system, graduate parents would illustrate the more abstract material with testimonies of their own experiences, thus enriching it for the benefit of all involved.

One graduate parent observed how their presence benefitted everyone, including the professional presenters:

*'I think the presenters benefitted and learnt from speaking to our parents, and hopefully our parents have left the course feeling knowledgeable, empowered and more confident in their parenting skills.'*

The participation of graduate parents diffused any fear that the parents had of being judged or criticised. This raised the credibility of the process and strengthened the engagement of the parents and facilitators with each other and with the programme. At the same time, the facilitating parents needed support, training, encouragement, nurturing and validation of their contribution. Some of them were still dealing with challenging and difficult behaviours in their own children. They continued to use the NVR tools to reconnect with their own children and provide them with healthier ways to respond to their behaviour rather than escalating.

 

# Learning points, findings and reflections

## The culture of poverty as an adaptation and a reaction of the poor to marginalisation and deprivation

In our NVR practice we are particularly sensitive to the lenses or the Social GRRAACCEESS (Gender Race Religion Age Ability Class Culture Ethnicity Education Sexuality Spirituality) (Burnham *et al*, 2008) – with the additions of 'Employment status' and 'Economic situation' that also applied to our cases.

In our specialist group there were a range of different classes, cultures and religions, among both participants and facilitators. Poverty was a particularly common factor in this group. In our meetings with the parents, we regularly came across and learned about the culture of poverty and deprivation, as described by Martín-Baró (1996):

> *'The poor live in a different world with their own norms and values and their own characteristics. The characteristic features of the family in this subculture, according to Lewis (1969), are that couples are unwed; life is centred on the mother, there is no childhood in the sense of an extended sheltered period, fathers are often absent; there is a strong inclination towards authoritarianism; and the emphasis on family solidarity remains largely verbal. Individuals typically have strong feelings of being outcast, impotent, dependent and inferior; they do not have enough impulse control; they are very focussed on the present; they are resigned, fatalistic'.*

Some people felt so ashamed of their deprivation that they would only meet us in a cafe or shop. In some homes we sat on beds because there were no chairs, nor even any room for chairs. This experience humbled us tremendously and made us much more understanding that the daily basics would need to be catered for first before we could hope to achieve anything else, particularly as the '*attitudes and values of a culture of poverty are being continually caused and reinforced by the normal functioning of the social system … and the social and economic structures produce and perpetuate it*' (Martin-Baró, 1996).

## Agencies involuntarily inflicting damage and pain on families

Most of the young people connected to the group were known to different agencies, and their parents were often struggling against these organisations rather than feeling contained or supported by them. During the group process, this relationship was sometimes reversed, particularly if presenters from agencies that parents had experienced as unhelpful before made themselves accountable and available for questions and suggestions and appeared to learn from the parents.

Many agencies often only get a partial view of a problem family, based on the specific task they are charged with, while we got a much more complex story. That is why agencies often do not see how psychological damage is inflicted on more than the person they are engaged with. For example, on one occasion the police raided the home of a family of Muslim faith early in the morning. They made the whole family leave immediately without offering them any shelter somewhere else and without allowing the women to put on their hijabs. This experience punished and traumatised the whole family unit and destroyed any remaining trust in the police and other public agencies.

On other occasions, young people were taken out of their homes to keep them safe and reduce the risk that they might traumatise their siblings and disrupt family relationships.

## Managing shame and untold stories

**How to hear and manage untold, hidden stories** of shame, loss, guilt, pain, isolation and silence and fatalism (Waldegrave *et al*, 2003, p91); while building strength, from a position of powerlessness to empowerment not born on domination and oppression but on developing preferred stories and preferred descriptions.

> *'The greater control persons and groups actually have over their present situation, the less convinced will be their fatalism'* (Martin-Baró, 1996, p217).
>
> *'Change in social conditions and change in personal attitudes go hand in hand'* (Martín-Baró, 1996, p218).

We witnessed that the shame of parents and their guilt led to feelings of alienation from their children and others. Parents often did not know how to reach out to them anymore and they were left feeling helpless and a sense of loss for their child. We also learned that many parents' and young people's stories had never been heard before, not listened to, dismissed, or simply changed into data, with professionals not taking the time to hear what they had to say (Waldegrave *et al*, 2003).

By sharing their stories within the group, the parents not only learned something, but were teaching each other, the presenters and us at the same time about their humanity. It was a very humbling experience to listen to them sharing such intimate, personal stories of their lives when there was no obvious material rewards for them to do so. We discovered that these parents, against all odds, possessed a lot of resilience. Even representatives of the public in powerful positions (e.g. the lead of the Metropolitan Police CSE unit) wanted to hear the parents' feedback and listened to them with respect and empathy. Parents were encouraged to ask questions of the presenters and tell them their stories, helping to break down the barriers between them and the agencies.

The self-announcement session, in which parents talked about what had stopped them being present and vigilant with their children and where they shared their own traumatic experiences, were particularly emotional and liberating. They were followed by a meditation on forgivingness: forgiving themselves and others and asking for forgiveness from others. Afterwards parents were able to access the announcement and look at their children's behaviour without excuses or condemnation, but with more compassion and empathy, which had previously been blocked by feelings of guilt, shame and loss. The meditations usually fitted to the themes of the evenings, but the forgiveness meditation was the most powerful as it often fitted with unforgiven shameful experiences.

In one example, we experienced the empowerment of a black mother of five children who had been in London for seven years as an overstayer, and therefore had no access to public funds. She demonstrated her persistence in keeping her 15-year old son safe (he was involved in selling class A drugs) by going to meet with her son's drug dealer in McDonalds and demanding that he let her son go. This mother gave a moving testimony at the graduation ceremony about this encounter and how her son returned home afterwards, was put on an electronic tag, and developed a more respectful relationship with his parents and siblings.

## Cognitive dissonance

> *'Cognitive dissonance is the psychic discomfort of an individual facing two or more contradictory thoughts that in some way imply an incongruence or inconsistency within the self'* (Martín-Baró, 1994, p155).

A cognitive dissonance can be resolved by changing one or the other of the dissonant thoughts through a change in beliefs or behaviour, or new concepts can be added. Family therapists call this concept 'strange loops' (Pearce, 2007). The group process enabled many of these cognitive dissonances to be unpicked and replaced with new stories and understandings. For example, young gang members would often overcome their feelings of compassion by justifying their violent actions with loyalty to their own gang and 'demonising' the others (Alon & Omer, 2006, p1). Another example are the girls who are recruiting other girls into sexual exploitation in order to gain respect from their abusers.

## Surprises

One woman brought her new-born granddaughter to many of the sessions as she was her carer. This baby became an important group member and a powerful reminder of how all the parents felt unconditional love for their children when they were babies and young children, responding to them even when they were screaming and required patience. The baby was therapeutic for the group and when the grandmother got upset and tearful, one of the facilitators walked around with the baby.

## Gender stereotypes and other stereotypes

We learned that CSE does not only happen to girls when we came across a 14-year old boy who had been sexually exploited by a 21-year-old man. We also heard about girls being involved in gangs. Sometimes the children and young people were doing well in school or were respectful, creative and pleasant at home (e.g. helping with housework) despite being in a gang or being exploited.

## Action research

The testimony given in public and the children's testimonies during the graduation ceremony were an important component of the course, a piece of 'action research', where the learning was put back into the community. Referrers, friends, family members, some of the young people and representatives from the community and the steering group (e.g. the police commissioner of the borough) listened to the parents' testimonies, gave their own feedback and gave the parents dignity, often transforming the way they perceived each other.

> *'I met other women there… I thought, 'it is not only me – they do have problems as I do. Because of all the skills I learned – I started to understand that the problem is me, without judging. Maybe she needs my help. So, every time I learned something, I used to go home and explain to her this is what I learned – so what do you think about this? To cut a long story short: I learned a lot and now I can deal with situations with my daughter, even outside my house. The relationship with my daughter is very good. She is very open with communication, which I appreciate.'*

Another parent wrote: *'It's a place of calm and stillness now, a real home. A place of safety... I have learned far more about my daughter and being a parent as a result of this programme...'*

## What constitutes change and transformation?

The NVR framework was meticulously planned but the outcome was organic. Each part of the programme was equally valued.

The value and ethics-based approach of NVR group work is committed to dialogue, accountability, persistence, mutual learning, reciprocity, inclusivity, liberation, freedom, wholeness and justice, participation, humility, love and respect and a non-hierarchical, non-oppressive, trust-building stance (Waldegrave *et al*, 2003; Martin-Baró, 1994).

A partnership approach aims to work alongside and with parents, collaboratively, rather than doing something to them or for them. We adopted the metaphor of 'weaving' the programme together (Waldegrave *et al*, 2003, p75).

The NVR ethics of partnership, persistence, participation, dialogue and respect enabled parents to open up. They did not perceive us as coming with an authoritative agenda (e.g. to take their children away) but with a real interest to hear from them and about their child. They felt 'looked after' and we encouraged them to look after themselves and to concentrate on what they could do for their child, thereby inviting them to get a different perspective on things. We learned that we had to listen to everyone's language and attend to our own use of language very carefully.

# Conclusion

We support the view held by Cressida Dick, Commissioner of the London Metropolitan Police, that addressing the problems of gangs, CSE and serious youth violence is primarily a health problem rather than a Home Office or youth justice problem, with prevention being a better strategy than enforcement (Townsend, 2018).

By investing in NVR as a national framework linking social services, schools, the police and the voluntary sector (as we did in the local steering group that supported our project), not only families would be connected with each other but whole communities. The NVR approach can become a shared language. This language is one of connection and good relationship-building, a language of respect for people's rights, safety and integrity, and a language of shared responsibility.

 

We would like to close with a quote from a mother who attended the specialist group and embraced the approach: '*I came to the first meeting with two black eyes and a heart full of sadness – I come to the last meeting with a heart full of hope for my son's future*'.

## References

Alon N & Omer H (2006) *The Psychology of Demonization*. Mahwah, New Jersey: Lawrence Erlbaum Associates.

Burnham J, Alvis Palma D & Whitehouse L (2008) Learning as a context for differences and differences as a context for learning *Journal of Family Therapy* **30** 529–542.

Clark L (2008) Youth crime soars in last five years as gang culture takes grip. *The Mail Online* **10 November**. Available at: www.dailymail.co.uk/news/article-1084549/Youth-crime-soars-years-gang-culture-takes-grip.html (accessed November 2018).

Firmin C (2012) Parents need more help to protect their children from gangs. *The Guardian* **24 July**. Available at: www.theguardian.com/society/2012/jul/24/parents-need-help-protect-children-gangs (accessed November 2018).

Hines A (2012) Royal Borough of Greenwich, Ending Gangs and Youth Violence (EGYV) Peer Review. Unpublished Position Statement of the Senior Community Safety Officer (Youth Crime Prevention).

Hines R (2012) Royal Greenwich Strategy for Tackling Serious Youth Violence and Gangs (10 – 25 years), Unpublished Strategy Report of the Senior Community Safety Officer.

Oldham J (2017) Gang members 'filming rape attacks on schoolgirls as young as 13 in south Birmingham'. *Birmingham Mail* **15 September**.

Martín-Baró I (1994) *Writings for a Liberation Psychology*. Cambridge, Massachusetts and London, England: Harvard University Press.

Moran L & Hall A (2011) British youths are 'the most unpleasant and violent in the world': Damning verdict of writer as globe reacts to riots. *MailOnline* **10 August**.

Pearce WB (2007) *Making Social Worlds. A communication perspective*. Malden, MA: Blackwell Publishing.

Royal Greenwich Strategy for Tackling Serious Youth Violence and Gangs (unpublished).

Townsend M (2018) Knife crime needs public health strategy, says London police chief. *The Guardian* **6 January**. Available at: https://www.theguardian.com/uk-news/2018/jan/06/knife-crime-metropolitan-police-cressida-dick (accessed November 2018).

Umunna C (2016) The government must get to grips with youth violence and gangs. *The Independent* **22 February**.

Waldegrave C, Tamasese K, Tuhaka F & Campbell W (2003) *Just Therapy – A journey. A collection of papers from the Just Therapy Team, New Zealand*. Adelaide, South Australia: Dulwich Centre Publications.

Walker P (2017) Knife crime up 14% because gang warfare is becoming 'embedded in our culture'. *The Telegraph* **29 April**.

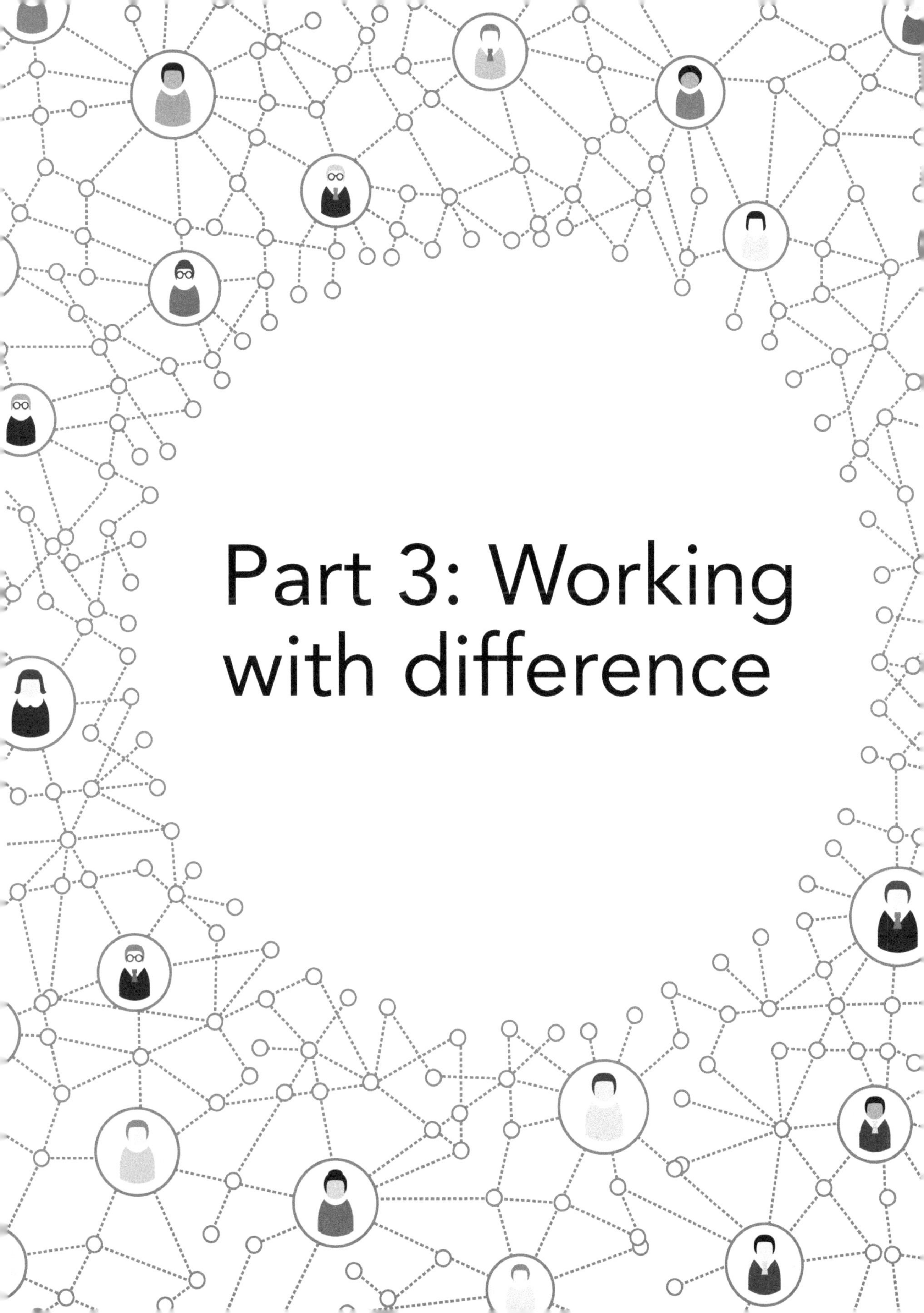

# Part 3: Working with difference

# Chapter 11: Rethinking the usual treatment for Black Asian and Minority Ethnic families

**By Julia Jude**

## Introduction

The idea of social justice is well established in systemic NVR practice, and to some extent it has become an integral element in many disciplines. And while it is clear that progress has been made in developing awareness of oppressive systems (Collins, 2016), the challenges of working with issues pertaining to oppressive practice and promoting equality remain (Maitra & Krause, 2014) for BAME communities in the UK.

Lowe (2006) argues that these challenges are visible in the inaccessibility of services to BAME communities and contends that it is an area that deserves attention. Why? All communities and individuals have a history that enables them to discover and make sense of the world around them in a way that is unique and different. But it could be argued that where there is difference in these histories between one group and another, there is the potential for unfair discrimination as it can create the opportunities for particular individuals and groups to be identified as different and therefore treated less favourably within the mental health system.

This is where the NVR approach comes in. The core principles of NVR are based within a socio-political context that underpins anti-oppressive practice and which encourages imagining possible future relationships through non-oppressive relational means.

In this chapter I explore how NVR can make a contribution to a more human and equitable society. Through a review of the literature I explore the marginalisation of BAME families: a marginalisation that can be observed in attitudes, policies, structures and practice. I argue that the interplay between colonisation and parenting is not an area that has been researched into. I draw on critiques of mental health services as a way of calling for a rethinking of how we work with BAME children and their families who are faced with challenging behaviours. I ague that a practice-based framework that is grounded in NVR principles offers an emancipatory framework that could potentially transform the experience of BAME children and their families from conditions of alienation and oppression that they often experience when seeking mainstream services.

Nearly four decades ago the 'Black report' (Black *et at*, 1980) highlighted the inequalities faced by BAME service users accessing NHS services but failed to identify ways of tackling the issues they recognised. Today, the issue of ethnic inequalities still refuses to go away. Lowe (2006) argues that we should pay closer attention to improving mental health services that are at present culturally insensitive to the needs of BAME families, and we should work to erode the idea that inaccessibility of services is anything more than an *othering* of BAME families.

Dogra *et al* (2012) noted that there is a need for better research evidence on the frequency of child mental health problems in BAME groups, service utilisation and, more specifically, whether BAME service users face barriers as a result of their ethnicity. They argue that a lack of evidence hinders future planning and policy, and that practice that could be designed to offer BAME communities purposeful and appropriate services. The idea that services may not be fit for purpose was highlighted by Holistic (2007), who revealed that BAME families and other vulnerable groups are not accessing Child and Adolescent Mental Health Services (CAMHS). The report recommended that CAMHS provide BAME families with culturally sensitive outreach support rather than with solely clinically based provision.

Not surprisingly, research and scholarly literature continue to highlight the ineffectiveness of mainstream provisions to meet the needs of the BAME population. However, this is not just about provision. Dogra *et al* (2012) suggest that even when BAME service users manage to access services, diagnoses are often dubious due to the use of a Eurocentric diagnostic framework that leads clinicians to interpret distressed behaviours, culturally unknown to them, in a negative way. Dogra *et al* (2012) argue that this unfamiliarity is harmful and suggest that, even if the diagnoses fit, racial stereotypes often influence judgements and assessments of clinicians and practitioners. This supports the observations made by Littlewood & Lipsedge (1997) and Fernando (1995), and is reinforced in Smith's (2003) report which noted:

*'Cultural and racial stereotyping is a common experience in the context of assessment and decisions concerning treatment. This may well influence the types of services and diagnosis individuals from minority backgrounds seek and receive ... and patients from all minority ethnic groups are more likely than white majority patients to be misunderstood and misdiagnosed'* (p13).

## Oppression: for sense making

In the UK there are policies and legislation that state that ethnicity has to be considered in service planning and delivery. However, what seems to be emerging is that there is currently sparse evidence that can be drawn upon to help deliver evidence-based and culturally appropriate mental health services for the BAME population. Lowe (2006), Street *et al* (2005) and Smith (2003) maintain that an understanding of the service provisions for BAME children and families requires a good understanding of the influence of oppression as a prerequisite for trying to make sense of mental health problems and service utilisation of the BAME population.

Making sense of our lives gives coherence to the things that we do. Pearce (2007) used the term 'coherence' to refer to all those processes by which persons invent and tell themselves and others stories that orientate the world around them and make it intelligible. It could be argued that the dominant discourse that prevails in Western-European thinking does not leave space for the BAME population to achieve a sense of coherence in their day-to-day lives (Dillard, 2012). Many black scholars have expressed indignation that BAME cultural histories rarely get reflected back in a positive light and they argue that they are fed an image of themselves that is tragic, misunderstood, wild and unfamiliar (Fanon,1993; Dubois, 1990).

To understand the world of the other requires a shift of perspective and a recognition of knowledge that embraces a polyphony of voices, ideas and discourses (Shotter, 2014). This is particularly pertinent in the literature on child development. Maitra and Krause (2014) note that the literature on child and parent social interaction largely represents the experiences of parents of European heritage, which highlights the issue of how culturally different values and ideas impact on our perception of parenting.

Otto and Keller (2014), for example, note that our perception of child/parent relationships is intimately bound to a Western-European model, which assumes to have a universal account of parenting. Carlson and Harwood (2003) suggest that the secure pattern of childhood attachment is often universally accepted as the single preferred theory for explaining child/parent relationships. Morelli and

Rothbaum (2007) note, however, that child/parent relationships, values, rules, expectations and duties are culturally and socially constructed and emerge to fit the context and environment of the society that the family inhabits. This is powerfully documented in the work of Takševa & Sgoutas (2015), which explores mothering in war torn communities. They argue that '*Mothering in conflict zones … emerges as a daily practice we term "difficult mothering" attributable to the pervasiveness of conflict and/or threat of violence permeating daily experiences*' (p4). The authors note that mothers' experiences of an environment where armed conflict and violence exists creates difficulty in the tasks of parenting as the need for survival heightens, leaving the parents emotionally exhausted and helpless, impeding their ability to care effectively.

## The impact of dominant discourses

All young people experience difficulties and established theories of child development are all cognisant of this (Lindon & Brodie, 2016). In Western European culture there is an expectation that young people will go through a transition period where difficulties emerge, irrespective of their ethnicity. However, research and scholarly literature (hooks, 2001; Maitra & Krause, 2014; Barns *et al*, 2006) suggest that BAME children experience specific difficulties due to their ethnicity, which adds another layer of complexity and stress to their mental well-being and family relationships.

But the nature of this other layer of complexity is a source of contention. According to Patton (2017), the 'other layer' is the harshness of BAME parents/carers' parenting style, adopted by some as an attempt to protect their children from the perceived ills of the outside world: drugs, gangs, violence, racist education systems, poverty, unemployment, sexual exploitation and radicalisation. Coley *et al* (2014) claim that this form of parenting tends to rely on physical punishment, well documented by Angelou (1969), Baldwin (1963), Briscoe (2006), and eloquently described by hooks (2016) who noted, 'like many adults who were verbally and/or physically abused as children, I spent a lot of my life trying to deny the bad things that had happened… In my case, the more successful I became, the more I wanted to cease speaking the truth about my childhood'.

## The relevance of history

A rhizome is a plant that sends and produces multiple roots and shoots. It could be used to describe the cultural practices, values and beliefs that underpin how children are brought up in families and communities. These cultural practices are often fluid, diverse and in a constant state of flux. They are also a significant factor in decisions about child protection, particularly for BAME children and their families. One recurring issue widely debated among practitioners regarding BAME parents/carers is in relation to cultural practices is the use of physical punishment (Williams, 2014). However, the use of physical punishment is not the characteristic of parenting for BAME families. Physical punishment is carried out by many parents, in many communities, countries and continents. Patton (2017) suggests that the use of physical punishment by BAME parents/carers needs to be understood in the context of historical racism and the traumas of slavery (Patton, 2017; Degruy, 2005; Hooks, 2001). Patton (2017) goes on to suggest that Europeans have a long history of being harsh and punitive towards children and argues that historians, anthropologists and ethnographers have found no evidence that corporal punishment was a common practice in pre-colonial West African societies before the Atlantic slave trade. Patton (2017) argues that corporal punishment in black communities is a consequence of slavery (Degruy, 2005), oppressive practices and discrimination that continue to erode the vitality of black life, and feed the dehumanisation of black children.

But it is not only about the child rearing practices of BAME parents and carers. Williams (2013) suggests the idea that difficulties in communication are an added problem. Namely, that many BAME families are not well-acquainted with terms such as 'child protection', 'child abuse' and 'neglect'. Moreover, Kai *et al* (2007) report that unfamiliarity often leads to anxieties about not knowing the rules and norms of the welfare system and law in the UK, which often leads to difficult relationships between BAME communities and child protection agencies.

Despite the above, the use of physical punishment is unacceptable at any level. The tragic case of Victoria Climbié (Laming, 2003) is an example of how BAME children can be made vulnerable as a result of practitioners feeling hindered by their unfamiliarity with cultural practices (Kai *et al*, 2007). What is important here is finding a bridge where practitioners and families can come together and better understand each other. One way forward would be to create opportunities to take into account the historical contexts of BAME communities and their impact on the day-to-day cultural practices of BAME parenting. This exploration could remove the too often predictable explanation that BAME parents/carers are simply unfit to parent (Williams, 2013), allowing for more complexity and better listening (Shotter, 2016).

BAME children are more likely than white majority children to be placed on the child protection register, removed from their families and come into contact with social services as a result of parents/carers overly chastising their children (Williams, 2013). Smith (2003) found that a '*high percentage of BAME children were subjected to inappropriate and inadequate intervention in the child protection process and in the most extreme instances this could be perceived as oppressive practice*' (p9).

## Cultural competency

Negative attitudes, beliefs and discourses about BAME communities are not without consequence. There is a need for mental health clinicians to become conversant in how racial trauma, poverty, chronic stress and internalised racism impact on BAME child and parent relationships. I argue that it makes no sense to have discussions about the mental health of the BAME population without naming the impact of history (Gilroy, 2013; hooks, 2001; DeGruy, 2005). Mental health discourse is socially constructed and thus services in the UK, more often than not, tend to favour a Western-European perspective on what is best for BAME children and their families (Williams, 2013). This perspective often clashes with the needs of BAME communities and may be responsible for alienating them.

It could be argued that clinicians need to be sufficiently trained to have a good enough understanding to ensure that cultural biases do not implicitly or explicitly operate (Otto & Keller, 2014). The importance of cultural sensitivity in practice was raised by Barns *et al* (2006) who noted that culturally competent practice is beneficial for children's well-being, but in addition that an understanding of different child rearing is essential in early intervention for BAME families.

A sensitivity to cultural issues brings attention to an appreciation of discourses that attend to cultural competency (Abrams & Moio, 2013; Nylund, 2008). Maitra and Krause (2014) note that culturally sensitive practice and intervention can best be achieved through practices that promote a cultural diversity that is accessible and sustainable within communities. I argue that NVR could offer a way of working with BAME and marginalised communities as it is anchored within a discourse that has an appreciation of community and humanity. By that I mean that the approach focuses on 'we-ness' rather than 'I-ness', collective needs over individual needs, connection rather than disconnection, and doing rather than abstract dialogue. An NVR approach is a deliberate shift from the Western-European focus on theory, which rejects practice that does not fall within its boundary (Shotter, 2016; Sousa Santos, 2014). Appreciation of practice that intentionally sits outside Western-European ideas can be traced back to indigenous discourses (Dei, 2011) and the criticism of black scholars (Fanon, 1993).

## Integrating post-colonial ideas into NVR practice

NVR could be more relevant for BAME families than approaches based on abstract theories and ideas that are detached from everyday lived experiences. I argue that NVR offers an alternative way of reaching out to communities in those ways of doing, thinking, acting and communicating; it connects with a discourse that is appreciative of lived experience as opposed to theoretical and conceptual ways of knowing. It is an approach that focuses on collaboration, reflexivity, participation and performance. It goes beyond words and traditional frames of talking about the 'worry', which resonates with a more Western-framed parenting approach. As noted by Shotter (2016), we learn to understand our responses by doing and not by looking and talking about it. Moreover, the idea of performance creates an opening for explorations of positionality, identities, beliefs and values which shape the stories told, lived and remembered (Pearce, 2007).

Below are some practice ideas that could be used as a way of integrating post-colonial ideas and NVR practice which could provide a fresh way of supporting the engagement of BAME service users and their families.

# Practice ideas

## Giving BAME parents/carers back their dignity

When working with BAME families, practitioners could benefit from placing the Announcement and De-escalating principles of NVR early in the training programme. BAME parents often make first contact with mental health services feeling undermined, labelled and attached to many negative stories of self, as evidenced by research (Chand, 2005). Not surprisingly, the feelings of shame are heightened (Weinlatt & Omer, 2008). It is important to give BAME parents opportunities to reclaim their identity and dignity as a way of showing a level of considered appreciation and sensitivity of their position, and to counteract the dominant narratives that they encounter at points of entry into the mental health and child protection systems.

## Creating poly-narratives: embedding post-colonial ideas within the NVR approach, practice and training

When the historical context of NVR is given it is usual to cite the influences of Gandhi, Martin Luther King Jr and Rosa Parks. This should, however, be reconsidered, because much more needs to be done to integrate post-colonial ideas and concepts into the approach as a way of creating awareness of the inter-relationship between colonisation and the BAME parental stance. For example, hooks' (2016) account of parenting could be a focal point of discussion. Parents could be invited to share their ideas while being open to the responses of others. In this way parents would be supported to find their voice to speak of their connection/disconnection as a way of supporting an emerging grammar of parenting.

Mobilising an emancipatory narrative from post-colonial literature alongside the NVR approach and training could encourage BAME parents to become better acquainted with ideas of post-colonisation as a way of helping them to examine their values and beliefs. This would support BAME parents to rewrite their parenting scripts (Byng-Hall, 1996) and thereby release the colonial 'ghost' from their lived and told parenting stories (Pearce, 2007).

## E-dialogue – social media relational exchange

Considering the internet's popularity and widespread availability, social media could be used to provide everyday accounts of BAME communities and their experiences of parenting.

Making use of social media to show the different ways BAME communities dialogue on the subject of parenting/caring and cultural practices could offer different pathways to exploring sensitive issues from an outer/inner perspective. By that I mean creating opportunities for BAME parents to explore and listen to narratives of parenting from communities that they are familiar with or have a sense of connection with. This dialogical social media relational exchange would be situated initially from an outer context, shifting to an inner perspective where the focus would be on the BAME parent/carer's positionality on parenting. This method of social relational exchange could help create a sense of ordinariness and relatability. Bhui *et al*'s (2015) study indicates that communication between BAME service users and professionals is often poor, leading to a lack of engagement. Moreover, the authors claim that their findings are mirrored in the USA, Canada, Australia and other countries with a European cultural heritage (p2).

The use of social media can provide much-needed opportunities to begin the process of improving communication and engagement, moving towards promoting responsive practice with BAME service users and providing other ways of exploring cultural differences, expectations and social understandings of parenting.

## Graduate parents

Encouraging BAME graduate parents to share their stories maximises the range of experiences and storytelling offered to BAME service users, thereby supporting a change in parenting responses and fostering alternative cultural norms.

 

## Reflection

Encouraging BAME families to explore the narratives of scholarly works, fictional and non-fictional writing on parenting is one way of exploring the meaning BAME parents give to the descriptions in the works of selected authors.

# Conclusion

Indigenous scholars have described the devastating effects of colonisation in all aspects of BAME everyday life to this day (Dei, 2011). Bhatti-Sinclair *et al* (2011) note the impact on BAME communities of a lack of teaching about ethnicity and race in social work and the implications this could have for practitioners and BAME service users. In this chapter I have argued that insufficient attention has been given to the interplay between colonisation and mental health services delivered to BAME service users and its impact on BAME parenting and mental well-being.

Parents/carers need to acquire the skills with which to create a good relational connection with their children. By acquiring skills, parents become more aware of how they are responding to their children, which can reduce their sense of helplessness and can affect how conflict emerges and progresses. This shift away from helplessness can be seen in the parents' ability to master the skills of NVR through performance and through witnessing the experiences of others. Arguably, there is benefit in making visible to BAME parents the interplay between colonisation and their parenting and how the complexities inherent in the legacy of colonisation affects their parenting styles specifically, and how this in turn shapes their relationship with child protection agencies.

## References

Abrams LS & Moio JA (2013) Critical race theory and the cultural competence dilemma in social work education. *Journal of Social Work Education* pp245–261. doi.org/10.5175/JSWE.2009.200700109

Angelou M (1969) *I Know Why the Caged Bird Sings*. New York: Random House.

Baldwin J (1963) *The Fire Next Time*. New York: Dial Press, Vintage Books.

Barns R, Ladino C & Rogers B (2006) *Parenting in Multi-racial Britain: Parenting in Practice*. London: National Children's Bureau Foundation.

Bhatti-Sinclair K, Adams R, Payne M & Dominelli L (2011) *Anti-Racist Practice in Social Work*. London: Palgrave.

Bhui K, Aslam RW, Palinski A, McCabe R, Johnson MR, Weich S, Singh SP, Knapp M, Ardino V & Szczepura A (2015) Interventions to improve therapeutic communications between Black and Minority Ethnic patients and professionals in psychiatric services: systematic review. *The British Journal of Psychiatry* **207** (2) 95–103.

Black D, Morris J, Smith C & Townsend P (1980) *Inequalities in Health: Report of a Research Working Group*. London: Department of Health and Social Security.

Byng-Hall J (1996) *Rewriting Family Scripts: Improvisation and systems change*. New York and London: The Guilford Press.

Carlson VJ & Harwood R L (2003) Attachment, culture and the caregiving system: the cultural patterning of everyday experiences among Anglo and Puerto Rican mother–infant pairs. *Infant Mental Health Journal* **24** (1) 53–73.

Chand A (2005) 'Do you speak English? Language barriers in child protection social work with minority ethnic minority households'. *Family Law* **33** 756–764.

Coley RL, Kull MA & Carrano J (2014) Parental endorsement of spanking and children's internalizing and externalizing problems in African-American and Hispanic families. *Journal of Family Psychology* **28** 22–31.

Collins PH & Bilge S (2016) *Interesctionality*. Cambridge Polity.

DeGruy J (2005) *Post Traumatic Slave Syndrome: America's legacy of enduring injury and healing*. Uptone Press.

Dei GJS (Ed) (2011) *Indigenous Philosophies and Critical Education: A reader*. New York: Blackwell.

Dillard CB (2012) *Learning to (RE) member the Things We've Learned to Forget*. New York: Peter Lang.

Dogra NP, Singh SP, Svirydzenka N & Vostanis P (2012) Mental health problems in children and young people from minority ethnic groups: the need for targeted research. *The British Journal of Psychiatry* **200** (4) 265–267.

Du Bois WEB (1990) *The Souls of Black Folk*. New York: vintage Books.

Fanon F (1993) *Black Skin, White Masks*. London: Pluto Press.

Fernando S (1995) *Mental Health in a Multi-ethnic Society: A multi-disciplinary handbook*. London: Routledge.

Gilroy P (2013) *There Ain't No Black in the Union Jack*. London/New York Routledge Classics.

hooks b (2001) *Salvation: Black people and love*. New York: HarperCollins.

hooks b (2016) *All About Love: New visions*. New York: HarperCollins.

Holistic P (2007) Thinking and integrated care: working with Black and minority ethic individual and communities in health and social care. *Journal of Integrated Care* **15** (3).

Kai J, Beavan J, Faull C, Dodson L, Gill P & Beighton A (2007) Professional uncertainty and disempowerment responding to ethnic diversity in health care: a qualitative study. *PLoS medicine* **4** (11).

Laming H (2003) *The Victoria Climbie Inquiry* [online]. London: HMSO. Available at: https://assets.publishing.service.gov.uk/government/uploads/system/uploads/attachment_data/file/273183/5730.pdf (accessed November 2018).

Lindon J & Brodie K (2016) *Understanding Child Development 0-8 years: Linking theory and practice (4th Edition)*. London: Hodder Education.

Littlewood R & Lipsedge M (1997) *Aliens and Alienists: Ethnic minorities and psychiatry*. Routledge.

Lowe F (2006) Containing persecutory anxiety: child and adolescent mental health services and black and minority ethnic communities. *Journal of Social Work Practice*, **20** (1) pp5–25.

Maitra B & Krause B (2014) *Culture and Madness*. London: Jessica Kingsley Publishers.

 

Morelli GA & Rothbaum F (2007) Situating the child in context: attachment relationships and self-regulation in different cultures. In: S Kitayama and D Cohen (Eds) *Handbook of Cultural Psychology*. p500–527. New York: Guilford Press.

Nylund D (2008) Critical multiculturalism, whiteness, and social work. *Journal of Progressive Human Services* **17** (2) 27–42.

Otto H & Keller H (2014) *Different Faces of Attachment: Cultural variations on a universal human need*. Cambridge: University Press.

Patton S (2017) *Spare the Kids: Why whupping children won't save Black America*. Boston: Beacon Press.

Pearce WB (2007) *Making Social Worlds: A communication perspective*. Malden, MA: Wiley-Blackwell.

Shotter J (2014) *Getting It: Withness-thinking and the dialogical… in practice*. New York: Hampton Press, Inc.

Shotter J (2016) *Speaking, Actually: Towards a new 'fluid common-sense understanding of relational becomings*. UK: Everything Connected.

Sousa Santos B (2014) *Epistemologies of the South: Justice against epistemicide*. London: Paradigm Publishers.

Smith J (2003) *Inside Outside: Improving mental health services for Black and minority ethnic communities in England*. National Institute of Mental Health in England & Department of Health.

Street C, Stapelkamp C, Taylor E, Malek M & Kurtz Z (2005) *Minority Voices: Research into the access and acceptability of services for the mental health of young people from Black and minority ethnic groups* [online]. Available at: https://www.bl.uk/collection-items/minority-voices-research-into-the-access-and-acceptability-of-services-for-the-mental-health-of-young-people-from-black-and-minority-ethnic-groups (accessed November 2018).

Weinlatt U & Omer H (2008) Non-violent Resistance: A treatment for parents of children with acute behaviour problems. *Journal of Marital and Family Therapy* **34** (1) 75–92.

Williams K (2013) *African Parents Must Know: Child protection and welfare issues in the United Kingdom*: Bloomington: Author House.

TaksevaT & Sgouta A (2015) How conflict shapes motherhood and motherwork. In: T Takseva and A Sgouta (Eds) *Mothers Under Fire: Mothering in conflict areas* Bradford: Demeter Press.

# Chapter 12: Delivering NVR parenting courses in multicultural communities in a CAMHS context

**By Emma Fayter**

## Introduction

This chapter examines the challenges and advantages of providing NVR parenting courses in culturally diverse neighbourhoods. The chapter is designed to assist practitioners in planning and delivering NVR parenting courses in culturally diverse communities. It describes how the NVR programme was used in a culturally diverse inner London borough and how it was adapted to be culturally sensitive to the needs of local minority communities, with a particular focus on the Bangladeshi community. It considers pre-planning and culturally sensitive reflections on the delivery process, including examples of how the facilitator team adjusted their thinking and their interactions with parents in order to find shared meanings and cultural fits. The clinical case studies used are composite practice examples. Writing from the perspective of a white British woman inevitably brings a bias of privilege to the issues selected and discussed, but advice from those from the Bangladeshi community was sought to help counter this.

Zimmermann (2017) refers to culture as representing the characteristics and knowledge of a particular group of people, encompassing language, religion, cuisine, social habits, music and arts. She refers to African, Eastern, Latin, Middle Eastern and Western cultures as having distinct properties that distinguish them from one another. She also makes the point that culture is a constantly changing and evolving entity. Lederach (1995) describes it as follows: '*I understand culture to be rooted in the shared knowledge and schemes created and used by a set of people for perceiving, interpreting, expressing and responding to the social realities around them*'.

## The importance of reflection in cross-cultural work

The use of reflection was key in delivering the NVR course, to ensure that we continually strived to make a good connection between facilitators and parents, and to strengthen this connection where parents risked feeling misunderstood. The expertise of the parent facilitators and our cultural adviser were essential in creating and maintaining this connection. Parents were readily able to connect with the often very moving accounts that parent facilitators gave of their struggles with their children and how NVR had helped them improve their relationships with them. This allowed parents to appreciate the value and effectiveness of NVR interventions in real life family situations.

The team used one hour pre- and post-sessions for the reflection process, which involved facilitators joining with parent facilitators and the cultural adviser. This process included sharing observations and considerations in respect of individual parents, such as why they might be struggling to engage with the course, or to relate to others, or struggling with group interactions and cultural dimensions. Supportive sharing also allowed the group to focus on how each session had gone, identifying where the process had worked well and where we had struggled, questioning each other's contributions, responses and assumptions. We used Neden & Burnham's (2007) ideas on reflection to create a culture of self and relational reflexivity. Where we identified difficulties, we analysed our understanding of real time conversations and thought about how these could have been responded to differently. Through this process we learnt to stay with apparent differences between cultures and to deconstruct them through dialogue.

We considered potential barriers to accessing the course that needed to be addressed, such as language and communication issues. In our first group, for example, two parents could not speak English so we had to allow time for presentations and discussions in the large group to be translated. During the course of this reflective process we became aware of many cultural aspects to be celebrated but others which needed to be challenged. Some parents of Bangladeshi heritage positively described cohesive family and community support, referring to the existence of strong moral codes of behaviour with members of the extended family and community looking out for one another and passing on concerns about young people to their parents. Others described less positive experiences when their teenagers transgressed cultural norms. They described experiencing the Bangladeshi community as persecutory, judgemental and rejecting, leading to a sense of alienation.

# Planning

In planning and setting up the NVR programme, we thought about how we could accommodate and embrace any differences we might encounter. We were aware that there was a large Bangladeshi population in the area and that our referrals for the first course reflected this. During planning, we considered the local community demographic. Inner London boroughs can be diverse in a number of ways: ethnically, culturally, religiously, and in terms of social class. Within the borough in which we worked, according to the 2011 Census (ONS, 2011), the Bangladeshi community made up 38% of the population, constituting the largest Bangladeshi population in England and Wales. In our first NVR course we had nine parents, seven who were of Bangladeshi origin, two of whom were non-English speaking, one Italian and one British.

We ensured that we had a Bangladeshi cultural advocate in our team to consult about any issues pertaining to the community that we were not familiar with or did not understand. From our pre-knowledge of the community we were aware that matters of faith could also be highly important in family life. The cultural advocate observed the Muslim faith herself and was able to assist us in understanding both cultural and religious factors relating to the Bangladeshi families we were working with, and matters of faith with families from different cultures. This all helped to raise our confidence as a cross-cultural facilitator team. It was important that the cultural advocate had attended the NVR foundation training so that she had a good grasp of NVR concepts and could communicate with parents about these. During initial courses, several cultural issues emerged that we hadn't anticipated, which required flexible and proactive responses. This chapter references some of our learning, it raises questions about how cultural myths become generated, how we understand them, and how unhelpful myths can be dispelled.

# Structure of sessions

Within NVR courses, sessions are structured to provide different experiences of coming together. Large groups are often used to present NVR concepts and share understandings in the wider, often cross-cultural, group. Smaller groups are frequently used to share more intimate personal experiences, though of course this distinction is not exclusively the case. Within the small group work, we encouraged parents to break into sub-groups in order to best meet their needs, for example, it could be with the cultural advocate who spoke Sylheti, or a group of parents with younger children, or children with additional needs.

We found that the NVR structure fitted well with cross cultural work. In the large group we actively encouraged the exploration of meaning and the appreciation of other cultures. Where different practices between cultures were observed, we related these to universal parenting values drawing out the underlying parenting motivations, intent and common values. This helped to debunk assumptions and dispel myths about the 'other'. Deconstructing the meaning of behaviour and concepts in this way served to break down cultural barriers and increase understanding between communities.

With parents who spoke little or no English, more time was needed for them to share their personal stories in depth, so groups needed to be small. In this situation we always tried to have two NVR-trained staff so that one could work with those parents who did not require translation and the other staff member could work alongside the cultural advocate with those that did.

# Programme adjustments

## Introduction of pre-course information sharing about families

On our first course the number of parents was small, which made it easier to relate to parents' individual accounts quickly. It also helped when facilitators were involved in all the pre-course interviews as this provided a more intimate opportunity to become aware of a family's particular difficulties and current situation. With larger group numbers this was not possible. In order to overcome the loss of this knowledge and connection we introduced a whole staff group meeting before the commencement of the course, whereby staff who did the initial interviews shared what they had learnt about each family.

## Use of action-based and visual methods

During the delivery of the programme we become aware of the limitations of verbal presentations and conversations, which could potentially exclude parents whose English was limited. We therefore thought about how parents could better access the ideas we were trying to communicate. Action-based methods such as sculpts and role play are integral to NVR practice, and because they are less verbally based we found them particularly helpful in cross cultural work. We therefore included them more frequently and also used visual methods such as diagrams and posters. This seemed to make the material more accessible.

 

The NVR sculpt exercise was specifically developed to embody the NVR key principle of supporters. We used it to enact a scenario of a parent facing a difficult situation with their child. Through this, the parent had an embodied experience of being in the situation, first experiencing what it was like when they felt alone with little or no support and then contrasting this with what it felt like to be in the same situation with extensive support. Non-English speaking parents were able to benefit from this experience as very little language was required. By witnessing the situation, first seeing a parent in an isolated position then shifting into a supported position, all the parents were brought together in a shared and powerful experience.

## Harnessing outsider witnesses ideas

Michael White (1995), the founder of narrative therapy, developed the concept of outsider witness practice. He described witnesses observing and giving testimony to the new and preferred identities that the observed person(s) was displaying. We adapted these ideas to support our NVR work. Within the NVR supporters framework, parents choose how they want to engage with supporters and community support. During one of our courses we offered parents the opportunity to talk about their experience of the NVR course with an MP who was visiting our service. A number of the Bangladeshi parents chose to attend. They spoke with him intimately and eloquently about their experiences, and of how NVR was helping them. The MP was genuinely moved by their accounts and congratulated them on their achievements and ability in expressing themselves. Parents experienced the visit as very affirming, feeding back that it had helped confirm that they were not failing in their parental role. In keeping with the impact of outsider witnessing, it had affirmed their preferred accounts of their identities as capable, present parents who were finding new ways to relate to their children, thus bringing about positive change in their lives.

## Modifying shame/programme adjustment

As the courses progressed, we became aware of the pervasive nature of shaming experiences and of the need for us to attend to these. Shame was often deeply buried, not readily recognised and often emerged later in conversations. It rendered some parents helpless and isolated, contributing to a loss of parental presence. The issue came to light in the supporters session when we recognised that there was something blocking a number of the Bangladeshi parents identifying and approaching supporters. As we unpacked the reasons for this it became clear that shame was a major organising factor. In order to assist parents in overcoming shame and recruiting supporters we realised that we needed to address this issue at this earlier stage of the programme. We therefore adapted our thinking. We did not make formal changes but rather kept the concept in mind as a facilitator group and worked as a team to support one another in recognising and attending to these issues as they emerged.

## Cross cultural work

Of the five staff involved, only one, our cultural advocate, was of Bangladeshi origin. We were therefore immediately confronted with the inherent challenge of how to focus on a specific community without generalising or making assumptions, which could be considered as racial stereotyping. To assist us in this we drew heavily on the Social Ggrraacceess framework, an acronym developed by Burnham *et al* (2008), which helped us to think about how difference is represented and how practitioners need to attend to this when attempting to co-create therapeutic environments. Pearce (2007) refers to the many ways in which differences may or may not manifest, varying between being visible, invisible, voiced and unvoiced[5].

We sought to bring these ideas into our course-reflective processes and in our supervision sessions.

We also relied heavily on our Bangladeshi colleagues, and our initial parent advisers who were both of Bangladeshi heritage, when considering issues from within this community and in questioning our views. For example, when describing my experience of working with Bangladeshi parents, I planned to write about Muslim parents, but modified this thinking after consultation. Colleagues strongly advised against this, highlighting the importance of distinguishing between culture and religion and the need to see these as distinct entities. This led us to recognise that parenting practices could be too readily attributed to religious ideology when they were often cultural norms. This distinction was very important in reducing misunderstanding.

Cross cultural challenges existed for both families and staff. Many families were second or third generation migrants, and a few were first generation assimilating into British culture. In this accelerated process there are often differences and tensions between generations, with parenting styles needing to adapt. This may be influenced by differing parenting styles in the national culture and by the needs of assimilated children who have to navigate the demands and opportunities of different cultures and differing ideas about how young people should conduct themselves.

5 Over the years the differences identified have been extended to include gender, geography, race, religion, ability, age, appearance, class, culture, education, employment, sexuality, sexual orientation and spirituality.

 

Madi (n.d.) wrote about using NVR with Muslim immigrants in Europe. She noticed that staff often lacked confidence in cross cultural working when NVR was provided by a majority professional group from the host nation. She suggested this could lead to avoidance or racial stereotyping. She proposed a specific rather than generalised approach whereby professionals got to know the particular culture of each family. She noted that this process itself provided a great advantage to the alliance built between the family and professional. We found that the pre-course interviews and the time given for each family to share their unique and specific experiences was important in aiding this process.

Omer (2011) wrote about the New Authority model in which he advocated for a more collaborative approach based on mutual responsibility, parental restraint, persistence and building support, rather than controlling the child.

Madi (n.d.) suggests that New Authority addresses the need for a new parental model in immigrant families. She notes that the gradual process in Westernised society of discarding traditional authoritarian parenting styles is often accelerated and intensified in immigrant families due to relocation, disruption, loss, adjustment and assimilation, which can in itself generate further tension. She referred to immigrant parents describing the authoritarian parenting they experienced as influencing their own parenting style, however their children expected them to parent in a more permissive Westernised style. Parents were often perceived as being overly strict giving rise to inter-generational conflict. Religious and community values were seen to figure quite strongly in this.

Maisam Madi (n.d.) outlines a typically patriarchal authority in Muslim families with fathers having responsibility and control over the family and being the distant decision maker while mothers are the day-to-day carers. Bangladeshi mother's in our first group confirmed this distinction of roles but also complained about the father's lack of involvement and wished to change this. Haneef (1996) describes this fitting with traditional Islamic teaching, which requires complementary gender roles. Abbott *et al* (2012) suggest that immigrant families hold on to the traditions and social conceptions found in their original cultures and manage their homes according to those views. Oznobishin and Kurman (2009), Trickett and Jones (2007) note the fact that immigrant children generally learn the language and gain an understanding of the local culture more quickly than their parents and that this places them in a different position within the family. This affects family relationships and the traditional roles of all family members, and can lead to a loss of parental authority and functioning.

Many complexities contribute to this, one of which described by Oznobishin and Kurman (2009) is role reversal in the parent/child relationship – due to the parents' lack of mastery of the host language, the child takes on a carer role for their parents when they act as translator, intermediary or advocate.

Oznobishin and Kurman's (2009) study found that immigrant children described being in a more dominant position in their relationship with their parents and experienced less family support in comparison to their non-immigrant peers. They also described taking on the role of translator for their parents' as a negative experience referring to feeling embarrassed, as though it was psychologically onerous, and of it leading them to perceive their parents as dependent and less capable. The combination of the mediating role and low levels of family support were found to be linked to low self-esteem in immigrant children. Jones *et al* (2012) also linked it to them experiencing higher levels of emotional distress.

## Cultural themes

When working with Bangladeshi families, some common themes emerged.

### Shame

During the supporters session, we sensed that Bangladeshi parents were reluctant to share much personal detail, which became a barrier to progress. As we unpacked parent's concerns, a new layer organically emerged that related to shame-inducing dialogues within their community. Bangladeshi parents often found it very difficult to identify positive supporters for fear that private matters would be spoken about in the wider community. Because of this concern it took people longer to build trust within the group and open up, however there was a sense of relief and containment when these issues were finally shared.

The fear of being shamed related to being judged by others as failing to live up to culturally defined expectations, and this was often associated with the concept of family honour. These judgements were experienced as profound and were often alienating and extremely isolating, and could come from within the immediate or extended family and/or the wider community. Parents felt that issues of honour and shame were more marked within the Bangladeshi community. This had become something of a cultural myth not only for parents of Bangladeshi heritage but also in our attitudes as a staff group. There seemed to be an acceptance among the facilitator group that matters of honour existed more predominantly in the Bangladeshi community. This was an assumption that we were called to re-examine.

 

When Bangladeshi parents spoke about perceptions of family honour, parents from other communities initially found it difficult to relate to this concept. Through dialogue, we deconstructed the notion of honour. This allowed parents of other communities to talk about their concerns about their family reputation and the reputation of their child. Similarities between communities emerged as other parents described their own hidden and equally shaming experiences of community gossip and perceived judgements. As a result, a shared understanding began to emerge, with facilitators and parents both becoming aware that this was not a culturally specific issue but one that crossed many cultures. This was one of the benefits of cross-cultural working.

These discussions highlighted the power of shame, experienced by many families when they felt that their children were at risk of violating cultural norms, and placing themselves in vulnerable situations. The overall common priority identified by parents in these situations was that of their child's safety. It became clear that there was a definite relationship between the effects of public shame, the loss of parental presence and reluctance to invite supporters in. Overcoming the effects of shame therefore became an important focus of our work.

Weinblatt (2013) described shame as being a powerful influence in conflict and maintaining unhelpful patterns within families, and described it as a very public emotion, which parents and children connect to how others are seeing and judging them. He described his public opinion interventions as an approach to modifying its negative effects, empowering both parents and children in overcoming the effects of shame.

The following are examples of how we used Weinblatt's work to inform our practice.

## Shame and supporters

Bangladeshi parents described finding it difficult to identify supporters. They reported being aware, within their culture, of shaming dialogues/rumours about certain families with similar problems to their own, and were aware of these families being shunned by the community. Because of this they were fearful that they too might receive negative responses from any supporters they approached. Naming and understanding Weinblatt's description of the shame mechanism enabled them to examine their negative assumptions and carefully test out potential supporters, thus giving them hope.

One parent had had no contact with her brother for years. During the supporter exercise she identified him as a potential supporter but due to the humiliation she felt at her family's and friends' responses to her child's behaviour, and her fear of being rejected by him, she felt unable to approach him. She was very sensitively assisted to overcome her shame and to make contact. He subsequently became a very positive source of support. Making the situation public and overcoming her shame became an empowering process that was profoundly life changing for her.

### Shame, loss of parental presence and ineffective parenting styles

Some of the parents involved described public shaming as becoming a preoccupying influence, leading them to feel either hopeless and despondent or angry and critical towards their child, both conditions which make persistent parental presence difficult to attain. Omer (1999) described parental presence as both a personal and bodily presence and saw it as one of the chief NVR tools in resisting challenging behaviours. He described parents actualising it when they behaved in ways that did not allow their child to ignore or intimidate them.

One parent's child was returning to an abusive relationship, struggling to see the harm in it and being drawn further away from her family. Her relationship with her mother had become strained. The mother was trying to control her and insist that she stay at home and give up the boyfriend, which led to arguments and hostility between them and the daughter would then withdraw. This interactive pattern had become repetitive and was very stressful for them both. The father had distanced himself.

Through working on parental shame regulation, parental presence was reclaimed. This, combined with the mother gaining positive supporters and introducing new reconciliation gestures, helped to shift their relationship back onto a positive track and allowed their daughter to move away from the abusive relationship. It was very moving to hear how the simple reconciliation gesture of having drinks out in a cafe with her daughter helped to shift the dynamic in their relationship and allow the beginnings of a reconnection. It was also moving to hear how this developed over time into a positive strengthening of their relationship, with the daughter growing to understand the concerns and intentions that had motivated her mother's actions.

# Trauma experienced by parents and children

## Child trauma session – difficulties in recognising children's traumatic experiences

In previous sessions we noticed that parents frequently struggled to identify or notice their child's traumatic experiences. This seemed to relate to the overwhelming and preoccupying nature of their own difficulties. We felt that immigrant parents could be particularly vulnerable to this lack of awareness due to the often multiple traumas suffered and the additional stress of assimilating into a new culture. Jakob (2018) notes a potentially greater vulnerability in ethnic minority families who have suffered racial prejudice. He also highlights other factors that contribute to their vulnerability such as the struggle to assert their cultural identity and to express their needs within the host culture, or the restrictive or excluding practices they face from within their own community.

We were also aware that child trauma was a potentially complex and alienating concept to communicate to parents, and that this complexity was also likely to be intensified by language barriers. We therefore considered how to increase accessibility to the topic.

One approach we developed was to use a poster exercise which was designed to encourage parents to connect with the challenges that young people might experience in different settings. It was constructed to go from the general to the specific. Firstly thinking more generally about adolescents experiences of growing up and the kinds of pressures they might encounter. Then focusing specifically on how they felt their child might be impacted. It used the Social Grraacceess model (Burnham *et al*, 2008) to assist in attending to differences and the Coordinated Management of Meaning (CMM) (Cronen, 1994) approach to consider the significance of experiences in different contexts. Using a graffiti wall, we asked parents to write their thoughts on the issues that young people might face, individually, within families, peer environments, educational settings, local communities/gangs and at a societal level. We subsequently asked them to think about their own child in relation to these contexts. We placed posters with these headings on the walls and asked the parents to wander around the room and write on them. They were asked to think of actual examples of the difficulties that young people might experience in these situations. This provided a rich source of shared material that really helped parents to understand the pressures children experience, and to go on and reflect on the more specific pressures facing their own child. It also helped them to consider the similarities to and differences from their own youth, and the difficulties they had faced themselves. This seemed to increase their capacity for empathy with their child and their current situation.

Because this was an active exercise and involved generating short descriptive sentences or words, it was relatively easy to use across cultures. The cultural advocate could wander around speaking to individual parents about their thoughts and assisting them with the exercise. Feedback was more structured and easier to follow than the complexities of a conversation or a presentation about trauma.

This exercise also led to a complex and layered dialogue about humiliation and shame. In discussing how young people experienced societal attitudes, reference was made to how Muslims might be perceived in today's society and how this could be publicly shaming. This related to the false association made between Islamic extremism and the Muslim community and how this could potentially result in experiences of racism. Although parents did not identify it as a major concern, they identified it as an anxiety or a potential concern, particularly around the time of any acts of terror.

There was also a further layer of shame associated with acts of terror that are falsely claimed to be undertaken in the name of the Islamic faith. These shame-related fears needed to be borne in mind, as, if intensified, could potentially become an alienating factor. Facilitators and other parents became more aware of this additional burden and society's responsibility to reject this construction.

## Dilemmas

Some cultural practices posed dilemmas for practitioners. For example, by respecting parenting practices that emphasised the segregation of the sexes we wondered if we were potentially colluding with a gendered stereotype that was inhibiting the positive development of gender identity, equality and respect between the sexes. When faced with such a dilemma we tried to respect cultural paradigms at the same time as questioning the effectiveness of parenting practices. For example, posing the question, 'Would it be more effective at keeping your daughter safe if you invited her male friend to your home or a mutually safe place, rather than banning any contact between them, which seems to be pushing her to run away and stay out late at night, thus placing her at further risk?' When framed in this way, most parents were able to re-examine their values and position.

These kinds of conversations fit well within the NVR framework and allow for parental approaches to be challenged and explored. They do not directly question cultural beliefs about gendered parenting, but connections can be drawn and priorities for change established, as identified in the small basket behaviours, and in connection with the parental value of safety. This provides for a consistent NVR approach and for parenting styles to be questioned without risking disrespect for another's culture. However, differences between the facilitator's beliefs and the cultural beliefs of the parents can give rise to discomfort, leaving facilitators questioning their ethical congruence and authenticity, for example if they feel they are not upholding their own beliefs on gender equality.

 

Exploring these issues sensitively represents an ongoing struggle to find respectful, non-alienating and non-offensive ways of discoursing. This experience can mirror the struggle that families face when parents and young people have to negotiate conflicts in order to try and reconcile their often differing views and aspirations.

We offer no hard and fast solutions to these dilemmas as we believe that this is simply the complex nature of this work, and that one needs to be flexible and responsive in the moment to specific situations and the particular parents that are present.

## Conclusions

This chapter was written following reflections on running three culturally diverse parenting courses, and the ability to draw general conclusions is therefore limited.

Integrating reflections on group interactions and connecting them to NVR principles and to culture is very complex, thought provoking and challenging, often leading to further questions and dilemmas. However, we believe that the use of reflective practice is essential to the development of good cross-cultural work.

Once the chapter was completed I asked a Bangladeshi colleague – cultural advocate Alimun Nessa – to review it from a cultural perspective. My heartfelt thanks go to her for her invaluable comments and feedback and also to a previous bilingual co-worker/cultural advocate who has since left the service, who supported the courses described and helped to shape our thinking about cross cultural work with members of the Bangladeshi community. Overall, Alimun felt that the chapter reflected cultural themes and issues sensitively and she recognised many of them from her own NVR practice. She particularly liked the emphasis on reflection and made the point that, in her view, cultural sensitivity was not something that could be taught as such, but was something that emerged through attentive cross-cultural dialogue. She also noted the importance of facilitators owning their discomfort about particular issues and how, through facilitator discussion, culturally sensitive approaches could then be developed to address the issues concerned.

There were some points where she found the terminology used questionable and I sought to modify the text to reflect this. For example, as someone from the Bangladeshi community and a British citizen she found the term 'host nation' inappropriate as it implied a guest status. She also felt that there had been a regrettable change in terminology from cultural 'integration', which she saw as each culture respecting and influencing one another, to 'assimilation', which she saw more in terms of *becoming* another culture and not an inter-mix of different cultures.

She felt that the facilitator team should aim to be representative of the ethnic demographics of the area, or at least reflect the diversity of London where possible, be that through a mix of cultural advocates or persons from other professions. She also felt that it was important that all staff involved should have the opportunity to attend foundation-level training in the NVR approach, but ideally at facilitator level.

In summary, the facilitator team was struck by the universality of parenting concerns and how well NVR seemed to address these. Our sense was that the NVR principles and strategies were accessible by parents of all cultures who were readily able to relate to the ideas presented.

There appeared to be many positive benefits to cross-cultural work. It served to bring communities together, helping them to appreciate and understand the various different cultural values and beliefs that inform parenting and family life. The reflective experience involved also helped to develop our professional practice and sensitivity to difference and culture.

We found much to celebrate in the richness and diversity of cultural experience and family life, and much that connected us in common humanity across communities.

## References

Abbott DA, Springer PR & Hollist CS (2012) Therapy with immigrant Muslim couples: applying culturally appropriate interventions and strategies. *Journal of Couple Relationship Therapy* **11** pp254–266.

Burnham J, Alvis Palma D & Whitehouse L (2008) Learning as a context for differences and differences as a context for learning. *Journal of Family Therapy* **30** 529–542 doi:10.1111/j.1467-6427.2008.00436.x.

Edilstein P (2001) Social work with Muslims: Insights from the teachings of Islam. *Critical Social Work* **6**.

Haneef S (1996) *What Everyone Should Know about Islam and Muslims*. Chicago, IL: Library of Islam.

Jakob P (2018) Multi-stressed families, child violence and the larger system: an adaptation of the nonviolent model. *Journal of Family Therapy* **40** 25–44 doi: 10.1111/1467-6427.12133.

Lederach JP (1995) *Preparing for Peace: Conflict transformation across cultures*.

Syracuse, NY: Syracuse University Press.

Madi M (Undated) *NVR with Cultural Minority Groups: Example of Muslim immigrants in Europe* [online]. The New Authority Centre. Available at: http://www.newauthority.net/data/cntfiles/239_.pdf (accessed October 2018).

 

Neden J & Burnham J (2007) Using relational reflexivity as a resource in teaching family therapy. *Journal of Family Therapy*. doi.org/10.1111/j.1467-6427.2007.00402.x

Office for National Statistics (2011) Census: Aggregate data (England and Wales) (computer file).

Omer H (1999) *Parental Presence. Reclaiming a leadership role in bringing up our children*. Phoenix Arizona: Zeig, Tucker & Co.

Omer H (2011) *The New Authority: Family, school and community*. New York: Cambridge University Press.

Pearce WB (2007) *Making Social Worlds: A communication perspective*. Oxford: Blackwell.

Weinblatt U (2013) Regulating shame in intense parent-child conflict through the use of Public Opinion in NVR therapy. *Family Dynamics* **38** 62–71.

White M (1995) Reflecting teamwork as definitional ceremony. In: M White. *Re-Authoring Lives: Interviews and essays* (pp172–198). Adelaide: Dulwich Centre Publications.

White M (1999) Reflecting-teamwork as definitional ceremony revisited [online]. Available at: https://www.dulwichcentre.com.au/reflecting-teamwork-as-definitional-ceremony-michael-white.pdf (accessed October 2018).

Zimmermann KA (2017) *Live Science Contributor* / July 12, 2017 10:12pm ET.14.

# Chapter 13: Non-violent resistance: a Latin American community version

**Gilda Flores A**

## Introduction

This chapter describes my experience of facilitating several parenting groups within the Latin American (LA) community in London, aimed at supporting LA parents whose principal concerns were their children's or young people's violence and/or challenging behaviours. I will describe the impact that the programme had on these parents' strategies and on their increased ability to communicate with their children and their partners.

The NVR LA model combined the NVR approach with systemic and social constructionist ideas that perceive reality as co-created in social interactions. This formed the theoretical base of the LA Non-Violent Resistance (LANVR) project. I will describe how we made connections between the NVR framework and systemic and narrative ideas to generate parental resources for action. Using voices of parents and children along with recent facilitators' reflections in a follow-up questionnaire, I will illustrate how the LANVR programme helped parents and facilitators to improve their relational reflexivity and their use of the NVR methods – changes that have been maintained over time.

## Context and conceptualisation of the LA project

I learnt about NVR during my training as a Systemic Psychotherapist at Kensington Consultation Centre (KCC) and Bedfordshire University, when I attended a training event with Peter Jakob on child-focused practice and reconciliation. I participated in NVR clinics as a facilitator and trainer in a Child and Adolescent Mental Health Service (CAMHS), run by Elisabeth Heisman and Elizabeth Day, and later in social care with Julia Jude in a South London borough.

My curiosity grew when, at CAMHS, I saw their manualised NVR programme and witnessed how the NVR method, together with systemic ideas, improved parenting skills and family relationships in a very short time (10 to12 weeks). I participated in NVR group programmes for several years with Julia Jude in social care as a NVR facilitator and trainer in a London borough.

After meeting Haim Omer and Uri Weinblatt at the first NVR conference in the UK in 2010, and learning about the 'New Authority' approach, I felt inspired to create my own NVR version for the LA community. I asked Elizabeth Day and Elisabeth Heismann for permission to adapt their NVR programme tools for my community. Being a Latin American women, a Systemic Psychotherapist and a NVR facilitator myself, I wanted to share my skills with other LA professionals to reach our community and to pilot an LA version of the existing NVR model. I thought that this method, combined with family therapy, could bring hope and strategies to vulnerable migrant families facing challenging behaviours at home but not receiving any professional help, given language and other cultural barriers to support.

The project ran three full programmes, with the first being a pilot project, where a film (DVD) was created to support the NVR methodology and to enable further group discussion. The project was hosted by The Latin American Women's Rights Service (LAWRS), supported by the Coplestone Centre and the Creative Therapies Centre, and funded by the Big Lottery Fund.

I had previously worked with migrant and refugee communities at the Refugee Council and in several other NGOs. I was aware of the existing social, economic and political pressures that all migrant and refugee communities experience, particularly those with a different language and culture that make cross-cultural transitions more difficult. People who make another country their home, as Clayton *et al* (in press) observed, have to reconstruct their identities in the context of a new home, new culture, new language and a whole new set of relationships. There is not a collective history that affirms and reminds people of their identity. The LANVR version was guided by systemic ideas such as the concept of 'relational-reflexivity' (Burnham, 2006), and narrative ideas such as 'externalising the problem' (White & Epston, 1990) in combination with NVR concepts such as taking a firm stance on issues of a) violence, risk taking and antisocial behaviour and; b) on the avoidance of all physical or verbal attacks (Omer, 2000, p48).

 

The programme, called '*NVR: a Latin American community version*', aimed to create conditions in which parents could develop their empowerment and resources to bring about change in their relationships with their children. The Latin American community living in London, like other migrant or refugee communities, face multiple difficulties such as isolation and socio-economic hardship. The programme was therefore created to respond to some of those difficulties and to help parents reclaim their roles as carers, in showing firm boundaries and in taking a clear stance against violence, while also supporting them to actively show their love and care, particularly to those children who were displaying challenging behaviour. Finally, the programme set out to create opportunities to deconstruct saturated negative narratives of identities into positive ones by organising culturally sensitive therapy workshops.

The LA community is one of the fastest growing migrant communities in London, yet one of the most invisible. In 2013 there were 145,000 LAs living in London (McIlwaine & Bunge, 2016). In spite of high rates of employment (85%), many experience exclusion, poverty and disadvantage in the labour market. Reports by Queen Mary University (McIlwaine *et al*, 2011; McIlwaine & Bunge, 2016) reveal that the majority work in low paid, precarious jobs, mostly in the cleaning or catering sectors, and experience 'in work poverty' and isolation linked to working antisocial and fragmented hours.

LA children in London face extreme difficulties in terms of school achievement, their sense of identity growing up in the midst of two cultures, while often having to assume the role of carers for younger siblings given their parents' anti-social working hours. Children quickly grasp the English language and often have to interpret for their parents at local services like the NHS, police, social care services, school etc, and as a result they are made part of adult conversations about social, emotional and financial difficulties faced by their parents. Taking their circumstances into account, the goal of the project was to offer support to parents struggling with their children at home. Either the children's behaviour was too challenging, or the children were experiencing physical abuse.

The project aimed to create a secure space for LA parents, regardless of their race, ethnicity, national origin, gender, sexual identity, abilities, religion or political beliefs, in which they could create mutual support networks and also connect with other useful organisations. The project used the NVR innovative approach that – until now – had only been done with English-speaking facilitators and parents in the UK.[6]

I was mindful that, in order to enable NVR ideas to be shared with LA families,

6 Most LAs speak Spanish with the exception of Brazilians, who speak Portuguese.

this would require a shared medium of communication and the LA pilot project therefore commissioned a film (DVD) to support the delivery of NVR ideas and to enable group discussions and role play to perform different styles of parenting.

To organise the project, I first delivered a facilitators' training for LA systemic therapists or equivalent professionals who wanted to participate in this new NVR pilot project. Once a team was created, we delivered a training for facilitators over several weeks. The team, in collaboration with other volunteers and groups from the LA community, assisted me greatly in delivering the *NVR: Latin American community version* pilot.

LA parents from the first NVR community pilot group came to a symposium on the International Day against Violence at LAWRS. During this event, graduate parents interviewed other parents and showed parts of the DVD, *NVR: a Latin American community version*. The symposium was well attended by the LA community and more than 50 parents were present. As a result of this presentation we were asked to deliver more programmes and to give talks at open days in a number of schools that had a significant number LA of children.

Currently, there is no project within the LA community where families can access therapeutic services, such as family therapy and/or NVR groups in their own language. The exceptions are 'Anahi', a counselling service for women only, offered by LAWRS, or the 'Telefono de la Esperanza', a telephone counselling line that primarily supports individuals in crisis situations and is run by volunteers.

## Systemic, narrative and NVR theories and concepts used in the LA project

The aim of the following section is to describe which systemic or social constructionist ideas were used during the programme and how the different stages of the programme were designed and carried out.

Latin Americans are known for their love of music, food and dance, and for their preference to interact in small groups. When there are problems, such as language difficulties, domestic violence, abuse, discrimination and antisocial working hours, isolating oneself socially becomes a natural way of coping. Feelings of shame are often attached to those difficulties, which often makes engagement with support services very challenging. In addition, socioeconomic difficulties regularly cause tensions among family members, particularly when adolescents are targeted by gangs with the intention of enrolling them in their activities. As mentioned, many LA parents are employed in cleaning, catering and hospitality and therefore work antisocial hours. This working pattern often creates distance in the family unit, leading to the 'absent parent phenomenon', sometimes resulting in loss of parental authority and prompting anger, frustration and challenging behaviours and violence among their children. It can also leave parents feeling hopeless and not knowing how to parent their children, as the 'old' ways of parenting have stopped working for them.

Conduct disorders, characterised by recurring and continual patterns of antisocial, aggressive or defiant conduct, often lead to persistent violations of age appropriate social behaviours and always have a negative impact on the functioning and quality of family life (Meltzer *et al*, 2000). The concept of parental new authority (Omer, 2010) can help parents find an alternative way between the traditional approaches that use strict discipline and are based on the old authority, and the new authority that gives parents clear hierarchies between adults and children, but that moves away from control and distance, helping parents to co create a positive parental connection.

Omer (2010) suggests that modern parents are facing a dilemma as to how to bring up their children, as both traditional parenting styles and freer, more laid back styles are severely criticised because they do not show the expected results, leaving parents feeling hopeless. The new authority must be based on presence and proximity, not on distance and awe (Omer, 2011, p1-4). LA parents and carers who came to our workshops, had experienced severe disempowerment. NVR and systemic therapy enabled them to develop strategies to re-author their stories of blame and failure into successful narratives of parental presence and resilience. As White and Epston (1990) suggest, marginalised groups tend to internalise the negative discourses told about them.

Omer's concept of new authority is based on, '*selfcontrol instead of control, presence instead of distance, persistence instead of immediate punishment, transparency instead of secrecy, a supportive network instead of a rigorous hierarchy and strict non-violence instead of naked force*' (Omer, 2010, p1). This new, control-free authority can provide a solid ground for parents when having to resist their children's' problematic behaviour, which then enables the children to start co-operating with them, rather than having to rebel against them.

When developing the NVR programme for LA families, I used theoretical approaches embracing systemic principles including multiple perspectives in working with different issues of parenting, and a flexible approach that incorporated other methods such as mindfulness, sculpting (Satir, 1983) and narrative theory. White (2005) believes that we need an 'alternative territory of identity', a safe place in which we can give expression to our experiences of trauma and its consequences. *NVR: A Latin American Community Version* became that place for parents, where they could explore and externalise, week after week, their multiple narratives and meanings (Epston & White, 1992) of what it meant for them and/or their children to be a migrant/refugee/parent, and experiencing domestic violence, feeling powerless, hopeless, anger outbursts, punishment etc, and to explore these issues from a distance, without experiencing an assault on their identities. The NVR framework provided a safe space to explore and co-create alternative stories and identify small but significant moments that could bring change. The DVD film assisted parents to start taking part in role plays, where they could externalise and perform different aspects of their behaviour as well as embody and practise acts of love, reconciliation and announcements.

## Putting theory into action

Narrative theory emphasises that our emotional well-being is closely connected to our values for living and for hope. Weingarten (2000) proposes that witnessing is not a passive process but enables the connection with another person, validating their story. We considered it the job of the facilitators to hold onto hope for the parents (Flaskas, 2007) and make the NVR sessions an arena for parents, where they could try and transform their stories.

Inspired by the work of White and Epston (1990), the parents' stories were represented, enacted, written about and 'the good behaviour' performed, so that in the 'doing', parents could take time to reflect about the 'self' and get feedback and encouragement from the group. This fitted well with LA culture, where parents construct the self in communal and collective ways, while the idea of individuality is not a universal notion, but derived from Western culture (Bracken *et al*, 1999).

Satir (1983) says that the primary goal of a therapist is to deal with family pain, which can manifest itself in the symptoms of one family member but often extends to all members in some shape or form. We had family therapy input throughout the LANVR programmes, which families could access for support. This therapy looked at specific areas of the NVR methodology, deconstructing language and meaning, as well as attending to other areas that parents experienced as problematic.

## The structure of the LA project

The process did not start with individual or group sessions, but at a much earlier stage in the recruitment process when enlisting families, which took nearly three months before the start of the group programme. I first engaged facilitators and other people to help me with the production of the LA film version of the non-violent resistance DVD and with the translation and editing of the NVR parent and facilitators book. They also helped with the recruitment of the families.

We then contacted local schools, LA charities, local GP's surgeries and local authorities, and we wrote and published articles and gave interviews in local LA newspapers, and on radio and television media. We also contacted community leaders and local churches. The local authority, in particular children's services, was offered the NVR programme for the LA families they worked with who had children that were classed as in need and those with safeguarding concerns. Friends and colleagues were also informed about the project and asked to pass on the information among their contacts. LAWRS and other community and local organisations referred families to us who fitted the criteria of children or adolescents with challenging behaviour, and parents who felt a sense of hopelessness in their parenting skills.

All the NVR group sessions took place in a church community centre in South London. They were collaboratively delivered by LA systemic psychotherapists, psychologists and special education teachers. The programme was designed to work initially with at least 57 users (up to 15 families), starting with a contact interview as an initial therapeutic intervention, followed by group sessions and additional one-to-one family therapy. Additionally, parents could attend up to six themed workshops alongside the group programme.

The workshop themes were:

- Migration and culture.
- Self-esteem.
- What do you call identity?
- What is depression?
- Attachment and disconnection.
- Domestic violence.

Workshops, therapy sessions and crèche provisions were provided to all participants free of charge, as the entire project was financed by different charity groups, and later by Southwark Council.

## Family and group sessions

The programme included three to four family therapy sessions (on average) which were run before or alongside the group sessions. They explored the family's aims for the group, the family's background and the nature of the difficulties they had been facing. Using therapeutic techniques to establish a rapport with the families, these sessions helped prepare them for the group sessions. Some parents needed to work on issues that were identified during the group sessions and were difficult for them to process.

The group sessions ran for 10 weeks and lasted and hour and a half each. Each session would start with a mindfulness exercise and we would then show visual aids such as the NVR Spanish DVD, showing role-plays to support discussion and exercises. We also supplied the parent workbooks in Spanish, which contained tasks that parents could complete after each session. Activities and exercises were completed in small groups, followed by group reflections at the end of the sessions. Two months after the main part of the programme was completed, we would have two follow-up sessions. They were offered in order to recap and reinforce the concepts and skills learnt.

Inspired by Michael White's narrative ideas and Satir's (1983) sculpting metaphors, we encouraged the participants to use new forms of communication, like making sounds, naming words, 'feeling' the words and making phrases to 'show' feelings about how the session had been for them. After the first session most of our session feedback ended in this manner and everybody joined in. Another important aspect of the sessions was the co-creation of non-verbal embodied communication exercises, adding body movements as performative gestures. These exercises assisted parents at the end of each session to give their feedback, to express themselves, adding dialogue and new meaning to our conversations. These exercises became very popular and everybody took turns. It became an ending ritual at each session.

Some key interventions and activities to support the programme included text messages before the group sessions, which we used to remind parents of the forthcoming session and encouraged them to attend. Additional telephone contact also took place, depending on the level of risk or when parents were in distress, as a way to offer extra support. Parents could also contact us if they needed advice or encouragement to go on. As mentioned, a crèche for children aged between four and 12 was also offered as a culturally sensitive facility to encourage parents to attend the program, because most of our parents did not have extended families with whom they could leave their children.

 

Two social events took place during the programme. A shared meal provided a special opportunity to socialise, encouraging the group to bond and to experience a sense of belonging within the group. Everybody was asked to bring something to share for the communal table. This was an opportunity for people to connect with each other and to talk about 'home', their health, resilience and their well-being, and it allowed them to get in touch with and identify their strengths and resources. The second social event was the parents' graduation ceremony, which was the ending ritual for the families, which gave them an opportunity to invite their loved ones to show off their course accomplishments and their certificates. We encouraged family members or significant others to attend. Grant officers, NGO co-ordinators, managers and community workers from different community organisations would usually come to be present at this ceremony.

Supervision sessions gave us reassurance and support, time to reflect about our work and the space to have a pause, to talk about concerns and to listen to our facilitators' needs in order to go on.

## The voices and testimonies of parents and children

Testimonies of parents and children (qualitative outcomes) were volunteered during one of the graduation ceremony events, when a number of the parents and children spontaneously stood up and gave their testimonies in front of an audience, leaving their notes to be passed on to the next LANVR group. The following is a brief summary of those testimonies, reflecting their learning and how their social interactions and understanding of relational awareness was helped. (To preserve anonymity, all names have been changed.)

**David** (11 years old): *'I tell all the parents to come to this workshop because it is very important. My dad has changed a lot – he is much calmer with me now, he listens to me, he is more respectful, we can talk. I am very happy.'*

**Maria** (9 years old): *'I thank you all, because you helped my mum and me to get on better. She doesn't hit me like she used to do, she listens to me and we play, our home is nicer, we don't fight, she reads stories for me. We are a happy family now.'*

Parents said the following:

**Ana** (a parent): *'I wish I had the opportunity to come to a course like this many years ago ... it would have helped me and my family ... helped me to become a better mother to my children, avoiding years of misery and suffering ... In this* *programme I learnt how to control my anger, that I do not need to beat or to shout to be listened to ... I learnt to de-escalate and to keep calm in conflict situations and to stay outside trouble ... to talk, to feel not so isolated. I felt supported and encouraged to do things differently without violence. Had I had this course earlier, social services or the police wouldn't have been involved.'*

**Carolina** (a parent): *'If I had this course 20 years ago, I wouldn't have lost one of my daughters. The government spent lots of money with solicitors, social services, courts etc, but I didn't know what people were expecting from me. I was doing what I had been taught to: if your child doesn't do what you are telling them to do, you hit ... hit harder ... The programme changed my mind and me. My daughters say I talk more and I listen. They learnt that things can be done differently... I have telephone conversations with family and friends (abroad), sharing with them what I have learnt.'*

**Juan** (a parent): *'I realised that it wasn't enough to be tolerant or patient to be a good parent. One, as a parent, makes mistakes that mark the lives of our children. During the LANVR project, I had the 10 most enriched sessions that I and my son ever had... They helped us to transform our relationship for good. I discovered that my son's negative behaviours were the result of my own mistakes and that there are positive and healthier methods, which are appropriate...'*

What these testimonies have in common is that parents began to realise that they have *control* rather than *power* over their children. All of them had stopped 'doing' violence, and their actions had a positive impact on their family relationships. These testimonies also show how the NVR practice framework helped LA parents to focus on behaviour, getting a better understanding about how to increase their relational abilities, skills and knowledge to keep their children safe in the community.

## Evaluation tools and outcomes of the LA project

Altogether we devised three sets of NVR programmes and, as I see it, part of their success was that we spent a significant amount of time at the beginning at our first contact setting up a contract between parents and facilitators. This contract included the parents' goals for their children and for themselves. They were revisited in the middle of our programme and at the end. The information gathered was useful, measuring outcomes, looking at changes and variations in parents' levels of self-esteem, support, mood, distress, depression and anger. Further reviews took place during weeks 12 and 16 as a way to continue supporting parents to achieve their desired changes and goals.

 

The following evaluation measures were used in this programme to assess families: the CORE Outcome Measures (CORE-OM) the Strengths and Difficulties Questionnaire (SDQ), the Goals-Based Outcomes (GBOs) and the Subjective Units of Disturbance Scale (SUDS).

The findings of the evaluation measures were as follows:

- From a total of 57 families, 85% of the participants felt less hopeless and more confident with their parental skills.
- 75% showed an increase in their self-esteem and reported they were less depressed.
- 80% felt an increase in their sense of belonging.
- 85% experienced less shouting.
- 75% felt they had more control over their anger.
- 90% reported no more incidents of physical harm.
- 100% of the families showed a significant increase in management and support.
- 85% felt closer to achieving their goals at the completion of the course.

All the data above evidences a significant reduction in negative behaviours, both in the conduct problems of the children and in the emotional problems of the parents. The same positive effects applied to the parents' perceived distress, evidencing better management and support.

## Follow-up of the NVRLA project

NVR embeds the idea of learning from doing, encouraging and appreciating feedback from others. According to Wittgenstein (1953) we learn through doing and action. Therefore inspired by this idea and attempting to enquire into our practice in a self-reflexive manner, I opened this conversation up to LANVR facilitators. I wanted to include their voices as well as their experiences, making our process a circular activity, enquiring about what they had witnessed and what they were doing now with the NVR ideas they had learned.

I devised a brief questionnaire that I sent to LANVR facilitators asking them the following:

- whether they are using any aspects of the NVR methodology, and if so, what tools they are using.

- when working with the *NVR: a Latin American community version*, which tools they thought were most helpful during the programme.

Their responses were positive: all are using certain aspects of the NVR methodology, for example taking a firm stance on issues of violence, speaking out against anti-social behaviour and completely avoiding all physical or verbal attacks. When referring to the tools, they named the 'baskets' (Day & Heismann, 2010), supporters, de-escalation and the announcement (Omer, 2004) as the most helpful to use in the NVR programme and in their current practice. The visual aids were named as a good back-up to promote the concepts of NVR. Facilitators reported that they are now working more collaboratively with teachers and community leaders and that they become active supporters, when necessary.

The parents who came to our sessions have maintained the concept and activities of supporters and de-escalation. Parents are in contact with other LA organisations, who offer support, advice and family activities. They know they are not alone anymore. They know they do not have to suffer violence in silence and many have turned fear into hope. The *NVR: a Latin American community version* is still alive in parents and facilitators, as the knowledge and experience has been widely shared within the LA community.

# Conclusion

The project reached parents from different LA backgrounds and nationalities, some had children's services, police and domestic violence units involved to help with their children's violent and anti-social behaviour. Some parents had come concerned about their children's behaviours or their involvement with drugs, alcohol or gangs. All the families moved from a position of hopelessness in their difficult situation to a hopeful one, and relationships at home improved, as evidenced in the data collected and illustrated by outcomes shown and the quoted testimonies.

As early as half way through the programme I noticed the parents' growing sense of belonging and empathy. Parents noticed changes in their child's behaviour too – more settled in school and fewer detentions. The families noticed changes in their behaviour – talking more and shouting less, as well as learning to stay calm while avoiding getting into heated conversations. They also demonstrated a better understanding of their specific difficulties as parents and as migrants and/or refugee parents living in the UK. Many exchanged their telephone numbers and met at each other's homes to revisit certain aspects of the programme, thereby acting as each other's supporters and forming close friendships. This was extremely useful, as many did not have close relatives or networks of support in the UK. Individual group members became familiar with each other and with the NVR concepts, collaborated and evolved with each other, moving from a position of isolation to one of empowerment.

At the end they even passed their learning on to other parents in the community who also wanted to make positive changes to their own lives and to the lives of their loved ones. It was moving to see the positive impact the programme had, the parenting strategies learned, the parents' ability to communicate with their children and with each other, rather than having conversations which were destructive and abusive. I noticed parents were always more hopeful when listening to another parent's story of change and resourcefulness.

And as for Elizabeth (Liz) Day (Day & Flores, 2014), our supervisor, she said: *'It was extraordinary to witness the ways in which the facilitators embodied the main principles of non-violent resistance in their voices and their actions. Liz will always remember the mother who spoke to Gilda, with tears in her eyes, and said, "You have given us back hope".'*

The programme did not achieve the graduate parents' subsequent involvement with future NVR programmes. We only had their input at the first day of the second NVR programme and at the Domestic Violence Symposium. Perhaps this was due to their work and childcare commitments. This is something to reflect on for future work with LA parents. In this NVR programme there was no possibility for training parent facilitators as there were not enough resources. Parents without a facilitator's training may feel uncomfortable being placed in a facilitator's role, which they may see as an 'expert' position.

I was deeply moved to witness the parents' achievements and their courage, and I am grateful to everyone who has assisted us in all forms during the process. Due to lack of funding, we had to bring the NVR programme to a close, however the parents' networking has continued until today.

## References

Bracken P, Giller JE & Summerfield D (1999) Rethinking mental health work with survivors of wartime violence and refugees. *Journal of Refugee Studies* **10** (4) 431–442.

Burnham J (2006) Relational reflexivity: a tool for socially constructing therapeutic relationships. In: C Flaskas, B Mason and A Perlesz (Eds.) *The Space Between*. London: Karnac Books.

Clayton S, Gupta A & Willis K (Eds) (In press) *Unaccompanied Young Migrants: Identity, care and justice*. Bristol: Policy Press.

Day EM & Heismann E (2010) *Non-Violent Resistance Programme: For all those working with parents and carers of children and adolescents with violent behaviours*. Brighton: Pavilion Publishing Ltd.

Day E & Flores G (2014) Non-violent resistance: a community- group programme for Latin American families. *Context, the magazine for family therapy and systemic practice in the UK* **132** p32–33.

Epston D & White M (1992) *Experience, contradiction, narrative, and imagination: Selected papers of David Epson & Michael White, 1989–1991.* Adelaide, Australia: Dulwich Centre Publications.

Flaskas C (2007) The balance of hope and hopelessness. In: C Flaskas, I McCarthy and J Sheehan. *Hope and Despair in Narrative and Family Therapy: Adversity, forgiveness and reconciliation.* London: Routledge.

Meltzer H, Gatward R, Goodman R & Ford T (2000) *The Mental Health of Children and Adolescents in Great Britain* [online]. Office of National Statistic (ONS) Surveys 1999–2004. Available at: http://www.dawba.com/abstracts/B-CAMHS99_original_survey_report.pdf (accessed October 2018).

McIlwaine C, Cock JC & Linneker B (2011) *No Longer Invisible: The Latin American community in London.* London: Queen Mary University of London.

McIlwaine C & Bunge D (2016) *Towards Visibility: the Latin American community in London.* London: Trust for London and Queen Mary University.

Omer H (2000) *Parental Presence.* Phoenix: Zeig Tucker & Co Inc

Omer H (2004) *Nonviolent Resistance: A new approach to violent and self-destructive children.* New York: Cambridge University Press.

Omer H (2010) *The New Authority.* Cambridge: Cambridge University Press.

Omer H (2011) *The New Authority: Family, school and community.* New York: Cambridge University Press.

Omer H, Steinmetz SG & Schlipe Von A (2013) The anchoring function: parental authority and the parent–child bond. *Family Process* 52 p193–206.

Satir V (1983) Conjoint family therapy. Palo Alto, CA: Science and Behavior Books.

Weingarten K (2000) Witnessing, wonder, and hope. *Family Process* **39** 389–402.

Wittgenstein L (1953) *Philosophical Investigations.* GEM Anscombe, Oxford: Blackwell.

White M & Epston D (1990) *Narrative Means to Therapeutic Ends.* New York: W.W. Norton & Company.

White M (2004) *Narrative Practice and Exotic Lives: Resurrecting diversity in everyday life.* Adelaide, South Australia: Dulwich Centre Publications.

White M (2005) Children, trauma and subordinate storyline development. *The International Journal of Narrative Therapy and Community Work* **3 & 4**.

White M (2007) *Maps of Narrative Practice.* WW Norton & Co. New York:

 

# Chapter 14: 'Was it my face or was it the biscuits?' Working with a family using non-violent resistance principles

**By Carole Payne**

Many of the children referred to the Child and Adolescent Mental Health Service in which I work have a presentation which includes violent or aggressive outbursts at home, at school, or both. In the current political context of limited resources and long waiting lists, parents and carers often describe growing feelings of helplessness and disempowerment in their relationships with their children. Many have been involved with agencies for some time and have not been able to make lasting or effective change following standard parenting courses or individual advice.

I was therefore very pleased when the opportunity arose for me to undertake a training course in order to become an NVR practitioner. Locally, some parents had attended a group, run by a multi-agency service, at which they were taught a new way of approaching their roles as parents, restoring appropriate authority within the family and focusing on a positive parent child relationship. This course would enable me to run such parenting groups as well as applying NVR principles in other contexts.

Haim Omer (2004), who developed the approach originally in Israel, has further developed his ideas, linking non-violent resistance principles to attachment theory (Omer, 2011). I was particularly interested to hear of the further developments made by the course trainers, Denise Wilson and Margaret Smith, who have added ideas on the unmet needs of the child (Golding, 2008) and the PACE approach (use of Playfulness, Acceptance, Curiosity and Empathy) (Golding & Hughes, 2012). These ideas seem to offer an additional lens through which to view the relational changes which may be useful for the family, and potentially create a richer understanding of the experience of the child.

There were several parents undertaking the training course who had attended the local NVR group. Their feedback and validation of the effectiveness of the model was extremely useful. The importance of the relational focus in effecting change was clear.
During the training course, trainees offered several ideas for the delivery of the model. Most of the trainees planned to deliver the model to a group of parents. We heard from previous course participants that meeting other parents who were experiencing similar difficulties was almost as valuable as the techniques and approaches of the model itself.

At this time I was working in a family therapy clinic and I began to reflect that the principles of NVR might be particularly useful to one of the families I was working with. Due to their circumstances, however, this family was unable to attend a group so I decided to offer an individual package delivered in the family home. It is this episode of work which I will describe in this chapter. I have changed the names of the family and some personal details for reasons of confidentiality.

Connor, 14 years old at the time of writing, had been in contact with the CAMH service since the age of 12, presenting with impulsive and oppositional behaviours. There were high levels of expressed emotion in the home and emerging violence from Connor towards his mother. His teachers reported that he had academic ability but was not compliant in any setting at school. The request from the referrer was that we assess for ADHD. Coogan (2012) suggests that when violent behaviour is attributed to a mental health diagnosis, there may be a tendency to excuse the behaviours, thus disempowering both child and parents. Connor has two siblings, Tina, now 17 years old, and Aisha, now 10. They live at home with their parents, Jackie and Michael. Jackie is a counsellor and Michael has a senior role in education. The family are of mixed ethnic origin, Jackie was born in Jamaica, with family there and in the UK. Michael was born in England, with parents from Scotland.

Jackie became physically unwell during her pregnancy with Connor. She now suffers with a life threatening illness and has regular admissions to hospital. She is no longer able to work. Millham & Aylmer (2014) notes that in her experience of using the NVR approach, there has almost always been parental absenteeism in the child's upbringing, whether through mental or physical illness, depression or imprisonment. Michael works full time and has done so throughout their time together.

 

When we met them initially in the family therapy clinic we noticed that Connor seemed to hold himself responsible for his mothers' illness – *'It started when I was born,'* he says, *'I am a cancer in the family'*. As I progressed through the NVR training I began to notice that some of his responses seemed to reflect an experience of intense shame in relation to his behaviours, although initially this was masked by many contradictory declarations of lack of feeling – *'I literally could not care less about any of it, the family, any of it'*. This fits with the ideas of Golding and Hughes (2012) about the 'shield against shame' that children can develop if discipline occurs with rejection, humiliation or anger. Connor increased his behaviours as a defence, experiencing his mother's 'absence' as a rejection, having a negative effect on attachment. This presentation also had the effect of alienating some of the professionals who had met him, making engagement fragile. Connor thought that he had noticed that some workers did not like him. Jackie's attendance at the family therapy sessions was sporadic as she was often unwell. She spoke of feeling completely disempowered as a parent, Michael had to take over managing the home and Tina had stepped into a role of responsibility for her younger siblings. We began to build up a picture of a woman described as 'a strong force' by friends, family and colleagues, who was no longer able to act in her familiar and preferred identity.

Michael presented as completely exhausted. He spent large parts of the early sessions gazing upwards at the clinic ceiling.

During the course of the therapy we had used the ideas developed jointly by Roper Hall (1998) and Burnham (1993 & 2012), known as the Social Graces, to consider all aspects of difference and how they may influence our actions. In writing about developments in the Social Graces, John Burnham reflects on the ever changing presentation of aspects of social difference which:

> *'Expand and contract, collide, become foregrounded for a while and then temporarily move into the background, faded yet always remaining present.'* (Burnham, 2012)

When considering the individual NVR work with Michael and Jackie, I was curious about those aspects that might be foregrounded for this family at this time. I wondered how much their mixed cultural heritage may be influencing some of their actions. During my work with Michael and Jackie I heard about some of the beliefs and influences from Jackie's family of origin, which had shaped her actions as a mother both before and after her illness. Both were able to recognise the positions which they had taken during the onset and development of the illness. Jackie spoke of 'clinging' to her position as organiser and disciplinarian, until she could no longer do so, when she felt that she had no position at all. Michael spoke of being very happy with his previous role as provider and 'light entertainer' (his words), which was the role his own father had taken when Michael was a child. Michael did not enjoy his new role, particularly in relation to discipline. He felt that he was not skilled at this and often resorted to bribery in an attempt to enable daily living to continue (which often included hospital visits and providing high levels of physical care for Jackie). This reflected the way in which some differences in their parenting styles, slightly problematic before the illness, descended into chaos once the illness struck.

I thought that the focus of the NVR work needed to be both in the present and the past. It would have been easy to hypothesise that Connor's current presentation was directly in relation to the effects on the family of his mothers' illness. However, both Jackie and Michael hinted that there had been some difficulties before she had become ill.

Having introduced the NVR model, its origins and principles, I spoke about the brain and neurological responses to triggers. Both parents quickly understood this and Jackie was able to relate the theory to previous professional training. They began to think about ways in which they might respond differently to Connor. Jackie found this quite difficult. She held a very strong belief that she needed to 'keep Connor in line and teach him respect'. Her own mother had advised her that this would be necessary with a male child, particularly as Connor was of mixed ethnic origin and would be identified as different. We spoke about relational gestures, which are not rewards and are unconditionally offered by parents even in the face of rejection by the child. These gestures, made from a position of care for the child (Jakob, 2011) are an opportunity for parents to demonstrate their awareness of the child's unmet needs. This is an example of the increase in focus on the relational approach in the non-violent resistance model. The concept of offering relational gestures was very difficult for Jackie to consider.

During one of the sessions that Michael attended on his own, he told me that he had been worried about Jackie's relationship with Connor for some time. He knew that she wanted to do the best for him but felt that Connor was only able to experience this in a punitive way. Michael said that he had only become aware of this since Jackie's illness and had found it hard to find the right time to talk about this, wanting to protect her from any additional distress.

 

**Michael:** Jackie's relationship with him hasn't always been good. She loves him, but she can't show it. Not in the way most mothers do.

**Therapist:** What sense do you make of that?

**Michael:** It comes from her mother. She thinks about a black boy... how to bring him up. It's tough, you know. Her brothers, one of them, got into a bit of trouble... Jackie isn't going to let that happen to our son. And her job, you know, she knows how life can go. And her mother was a strong fierce woman too. Not a hug, a stern word. Tough love.

**Therapist:** What do you think about that?

**Michael:** My mother was soft as butter, you know, too soft really. But we loved it. I have thought, you know, maybe we're not quite hitting the mark here. I should have talked to her before but, well, by the time I thought about it she was really, really ill. She had enough to deal with.

He had also noticed that several of Jackie's female friends had 'taken up the baton' for her when she had been in hospital, stepping into a 'strong woman' role with Connor. Michael felt concerned that Connor was rarely if ever experiencing the 'softer side' of a mother. I asked Michael if he would be happy for me to bring this subject into our conversation the next time that Jackie was able to attend, to which he agreed.

At the beginning of the next session, which began with me asking how the week had been, Michael was very keen to let me know that he had been using de-escalation strategies with some effect. This was good news and I wondered whether our conversation at the last session about Jackie's responses had in some way enabled him to reflect more on his own actions and responses. His body language was much more positive, I thought, and this fitted with Omer's (2011) idea that a person begins to radiate authority as they sense it in themselves.

I was able to move on to talk about Michael's thoughts from the previous session. Jackie acknowledged that she had deliberately taken up this position with her son, in accordance with the beliefs of her culture and her family. We spoke again about relational gestures and I used several examples which had been given by other parents and also showed Michael and Jackie the film clip of the 'Still Face Experiment' (Tronick, 1975). This clip shows a babies distressed response when a parent withdraws their attention. This had a powerful effect on both parents, Jackie in particular. She felt that this was effectively what she had been doing with Connor.

**Jackie:** [tearful] That's me, that face. I think, you know, I have been turning away from him like that. I haven't, not really, but he thinks I have. All he sees of me is that face, the one that is looking like business...

**Therapist:** What would you like him to see in your face?

**Jackie:** I want him to be like that baby, to be relieved that I'm there for him, to break into that massive smile.

We began to explore other ways in which she might communicate with him, while still being able to have some authority. I was able to refer back to a previous conversation about the NVR approach – a New Authority. This time the words had more meaning for Jackie. The session, which had been quite emotional, concluded with Jackie thoughtful about what she might try.

At the next session Jackie was excited to tell me that she had made a relational gesture to Connor, feeling very nervous and afraid of rejection. When Connor came in from school she had resisted the temptation to grill him about his behaviour that day and instead had let him know that she was watching his favourite television programme and would like him to watch with her. Tea and biscuits were also on offer. The offer was taken up and a calmer atmosphere persisted for the rest of the evening.

**Therapist:** You said you had something to tell me?

**Jackie:** Yes, oh yes. The next day after our last meeting, I thought, what am I going to do? So when he came in, I said, well I'm watching EastEnders and I'd like it if you watched it with me. And he looked, like, "what?!" Because normally I'd say, so what have you got to tell me about school today? Because I'll find out, you know. And my face would be like [demonstrates an angry face]. So I smile at him and he looks at me like, you alright? Then he went upstairs and I thought, he's not going to... and my heart's going. But I got the tea and the custard creams and I sat there. And I turned it up a bit and I don't know if he heard it but anyway he came. He sat down and he stayed!

**Therapist:** That sounds good. What was that like for you?

**Jackie:** Oh well, amazing. I just thought well, goes to show. Was it the biscuits or was it my face? [Laughs]

**Therapist:** Were you there, Michael? What was the effect for you?

**Michael:** [Smiling broadly] It was a mellow evening...

 

I was pleased with this outcome, which was the beginning of some positive changes for the family in spite of an uncertain future in terms of Jackie's health.

In conclusion, I reflect that this was a complex case in which consideration of the family's ethnicity and cultural beliefs was important. Linking the effect of these beliefs with the introduction of relational gestures enabled the family to begin to make changes in their communication patterns.

## References

Burnham J (1993) Systemic supervision: the evolution of reflexivity in the context of the supervisory relationship. *Human Systems* **4** (Special issue, 3 & 4) 349–381.

Burnham J (2012) Developments in Social GRRRAAACCEEESSS: visible: invisible and unvoiced. In: I Krause (ed). *Culture and Reflexivity in Systemic Psychotherapy: Mutual perspectives*. London, Karnac.

Coogan D (2012) Marking the boundaries: when troublesome becomes abusive and children cross a line in family violence. *Journal of the Family Therapy Association of Ireland* 74–85.

Golding KS (2008) *Nurturing Attachments: Supporting children who are fostered or adopted*. London: Jessica Kingsley.

Golding KS & Hughes A (2012) *Creating Loving Attachments: Parenting with PACE to nurture confidence and security in the troubled child*. London: Jessica Kingsley.

Jakob P (2011) Re-connecting parents and young people with serious behaviour problems – child focused practice and reconciliation work in non- violent resistance therapy. *New Authority Network International*.

Millham A & Aylmer R (2014) Love Bomb as acts of resistance: Reflections on non-violent practice. An interview with Rachel Aylmer by Alex Millham. *Context*, **132** p7 – 8.

Omer H (2004) *Non-Violent Resistance: A New Approach to Violent and Self-destructive children*. Cambridge: Cambridge University Press.

Omer H (2011) The 'anchoring function' of attachment – feeling safe as the child of 'strong parents. Workshop presentation for the conference. *Beyond Behaviour*. London.

Roper-Hall A (1998) Working systemically with older people and their families who "have come to grief". In: P Sutcliffe, G Tufnell and U Cornish (Eds.) *Working with the Dying and Bereaved*. London: Macmillan.

Tronick E, Adamson LB, Als H & Brazelton TB (1975) Infant emotions in normal and pertubated interactions. *Paper presented at the biennial meeting of the Society for Research in Child Development*. Denver, CO.

Wilson D & Smith M (2014) The unmet needs of the child in non-violent resistance: Integrating developmental-dyadic-psychotherapy approaches – lessons from working with adoptive families. *Context* **132** p22–26.

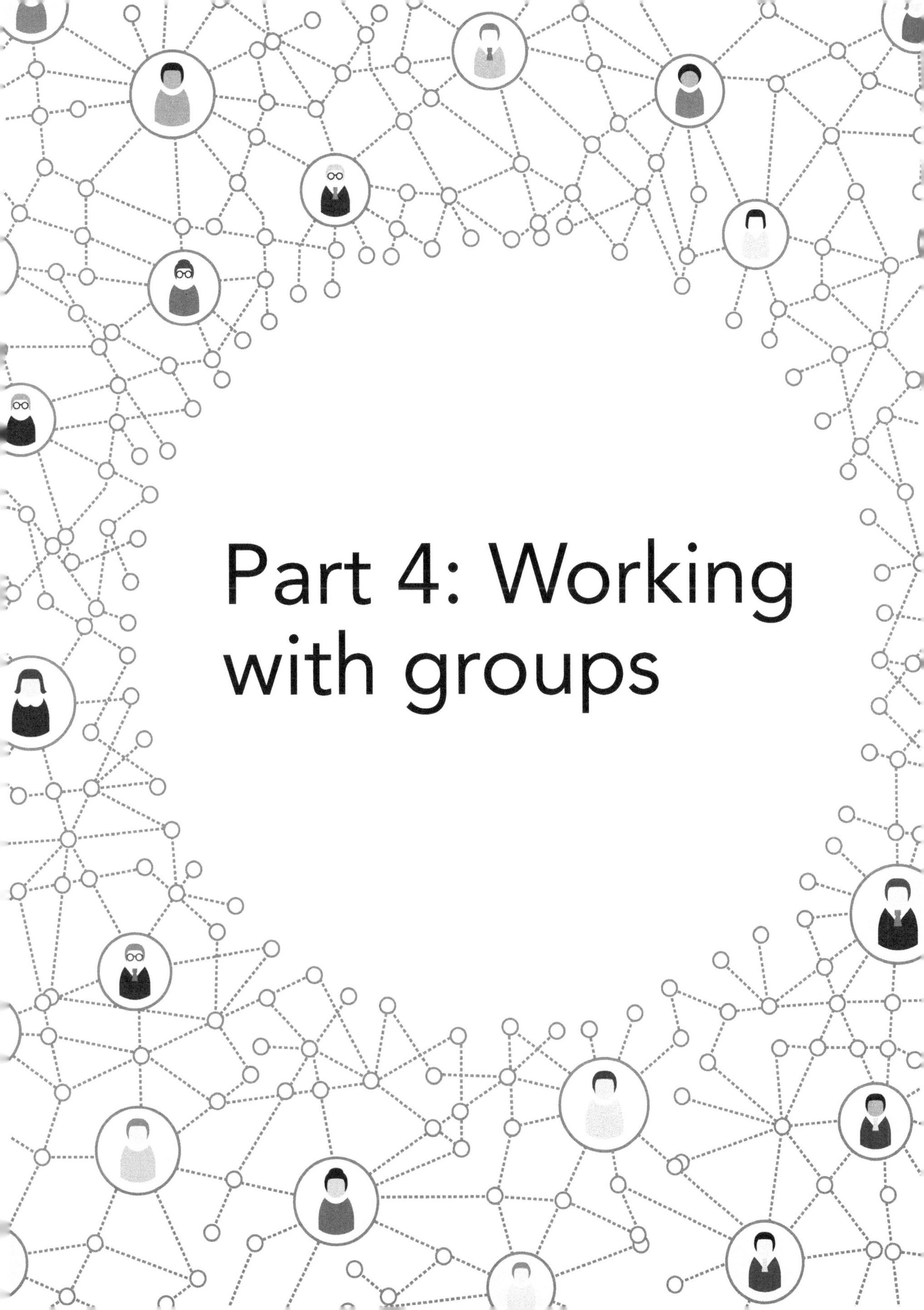

# Part 4: Working with groups

# Chapter 15: No group is the same: locating NVR as a group intervention within the history of group work, multiple family therapy and parenting programmes

**By Liz Day**

## Introduction

In this chapter I locate non-violent resistance (NVR) within the development of groupwork generally, as well as within the range of parenting group interventions that are recommended by the Department for Education for the parents of children with conduct problems. I show why NVR is better located within multiple family therapy (also known as multi-family therapy) rather than within parenting groups. I argue that systemic practitioner process research is better suited to understanding the value of NVR groupwork than standard outcome research.

## No group is the same

When we wrote the NVR group manual in 2010 (Day & Heismann), we were concerned that this 'manualisation' might fix the way in which people carried out the practice of NVR. We wanted facilitators to use our manual as a guide to the NVR tools and group interventions we had developed, rather than as a strict template that prescribes exactly when and how each part should happen.

> *'No man ever steps in the same river twice, for it isn't the same river and he isn't the same man'*
> (often attributed to Heraclitus, a Greek philosopher from the first century BCE)

One of the features of a group intervention is that every group is made up not only of the individuals who attend (and of course that will differ from session to session) but also of the stories, relationships, experiences, beliefs, culture, hopes and fears that each person brings with them. Additionally, 'stuff' (Shotter, 2016) happens in groups between the people who are in the room, and this includes the facilitators, who also bring their own stories, relationships, experiences, beliefs, culture, hopes and fears to the mix. The conversations that take place between people affect and change what happens in the group, and what meanings get made. There are also other internal conversations that go on and affect what happens but which are not visible. For example, how a participant responds may depend on what their experience has been of being listened to in the past, or in that group. They may tell themselves that their story is not as bad as other people's, so they may stay quiet, or they may remember being blamed by someone when they spoke about their child's behaviour and therefore censor their story. None of this conversation, which goes on inside the person, is available to the rest of the group, but it is part of what is going on.

This is a systemic social constructionist (Burr, 1995; Gergen, 2001; 2009; McNamee & Gergen, 1992; Shotter, 2012; 2016) way of thinking about people and what happens between them. It helps us think about how we orientate ourselves towards working with groups and how we act in moment-to-moment interactions. It is the fundamental premise on which our NVR manual was developed. These ideas owe much to the work of Bateson (1973; 1979), Maturana and Varela (1980) and Wittgenstein (1953). Later in this chapter I explain why I believe that the more usual *outcome research* cannot tell us much about what goes on in our groups and why we should use *process research* as well.

## Group programmes and group therapy

In considering the development of NVR as a group intervention (Day & Heismann, 2010), it is important to understand the history of groupwork as a therapeutic intervention in the UK and elsewhere.

Working with people in groups began with the ragged school movement, boys' and girls' clubs, settlements, and adult education (Smith, 2004). Groupwork as psychotherapy emerged in the 1900s when it was found to be effective in the treatment of patients with tuberculosis (Pratt, 1905) and, later, those with psychological difficulties related to trauma experienced during World War II. In the 1940s and 1950s the work of Bion (1961) with groups at the Tavistock clinic led to what became known as the Tavistock model (Hayden & Molenkamp, 2002), which is one of the three main psychodynamic group psychotherapy models, along with the interpersonal and group analytic models (Montgomery, 2002).

Groupwork is an effective intervention in social work and therapy and can empower marginalised people and communities to harness their abilities in order to bring about change (Furman *et al*, 2009; Kurland & Salmon, 1993; Preston-Shoot, 2007; Yalom & Lesczc, 2005).

I want to locate the NVR group therapy programme within this wider field of therapeutic groups, rather than within the narrower field of parenting programmes. This is because the intent of the NVR programme is therapeutic change rather than behaviour modification. Furthermore, we are working with the parents of children with significant mental health difficulties. In the next section I shall describe briefly the various types of parenting programme, before showing why I think our programme has a better fit with a multi-family or multiple family therapy approach.

## Parenting programmes

A number of group parenting programmes are used to address behavioural problems in children. The best known, with the largest evidence base (dating back more than 30 years), are The Incredible Years and the Positive Parenting Program (Triple P). The Incredible Years was developed in the US by Carolyn Webster-Stratton (2009; 2013). Triple P was developed in Australia. Both are widely used in the UK and in a number of other Western countries, as well as in cities such as Hong Kong and Singapore, which have significant Western influence. The programmes' main aims are to change the child's behaviour, help the child develop self-regulation, and empower and educate the parents.

The Department for Education (DfE) Commissioning Toolkit lists 51 parenting interventions and uses a star rating system to indicate the effectiveness of each. This star rating is based on the outcome of research trials. The more trials the better, especially if they are randomised control trials. The longer the programme has been in use the more research there will have been and the number of stars is likely to be higher.

On its website, the DfE said:

*'All of the interventions listed here have some objective evidence of consistently improving outcomes for parents and children. This means that the parenting programme has undergone an evaluation that has:*

- *observed a statistically significant positive change in one child outcome or one parent/child outcome*
- *observed this change with standardised measures completed by the parents before and after participating in the programme*
- *observed this change with at least 20 families representative of the target population*
- *observed no negative changes in the parents' or child's behaviour.'*

The website is no longer available and has been replaced by the *Commissioning Toolkit of Parenting Programmes* hosted by the Social Care Institute for Excellence with a searchable database of over 100 parenting interventions (https://www.scie-socialcareonline.org.uk/commissioning-toolkit-of-parenting-programmes/r/a11G0000001801sIAA).

Any programme that helps parents understand their child's development and encourages them to adopt acceptable and nurturing strategies for managing behaviour is likely to have positive outcomes. An intervention that brings parents together in a safe setting to share their experiences and offers appropriate advice on child care will reduce isolation, engender support and make people feel better (Asen & Scholz, 2010). This is the basis on which many long-established organisations for parents have been built and have thrived. The DfE rightly emphasises that a parenting programme that advocates a punitive approach, or which fails to connect with child development theory, can have a damaging effect.

NVR is currently being considered for inclusion in the DfE's Commissioning Toolkit. The Toolkit covers a range of parenting interventions that fall into four main groups, with some overlaps. Group one is general parenting programmes (the Solihull Approach Parenting Group (Appleton *et al*, 2016) and Raising Children, Family Foundations). Group two is programmes for behavioural difficulties (The Incredible Years, Triple P, Take 3, Mellow Parenting (Macbeth *et al*, 2015; Thomson *et al*, 2014)). Group three is programmes targeted at particular types of family (mothers and infants in prison, children on a child protection plan, children with attention deficit hyperactivity disorder (ADHD) and children with learning difficulties). Group four is intensive programmes targeting more extreme antisocial and offending behaviour (functional family therapy (FFT), multi-systemic therapy (MST), mentalisation-based treatment for families and multi-dimensional treatment foster care (MTFC)). Group four also includes programmes targeting specific groups (children who sexually abuse others, children who have been abused, young people who misuse substances and children in foster care). This list is constantly being added to as more specialist programmes are developed.

The parenting programmes in groups one, two and three are mainly group interventions, whereas the programmes in group four are delivered to individuals and their families by teams of workers, and are therefore costly to deliver. Interventions in group four have a strong systemic basis and were developed by therapists working with the whole family.

The DfE (2012) promotes intensive, cost-effective and evidence-based interventions for looked-after children and children on the edge of care or custody: FFT, MST, MTFC, and Keeping Foster and Kinship Carers Safe and Supported, which is based on MTFC principles.

Several community-based parenting programmes are currently in use in the UK, and more may well be in development. The main ones are Strengthening Families Strengthening Communities (Steele *et al*, 2000) developed by the Race Equality Foundation, and Empowering Parents Empowering Communities (Day *et al*, 2012a; 2012b). Family Action have developed Parents as Partners, an eight-week course for parents available in some London boroughs. None of these courses targets parents whose children are displaying significant violence or behaviours that are controlling or extreme.

## Multiple family therapy

The NVR therapy programme has more in common with multiple family therapy than with a traditional parenting programme, because it is a therapeutic group intervention based on systemic principles.

Multiple family therapy is an established way of working with families in a group. The approach emerged in the US in the 1940s and 1950s. Peter Laqueur (1972) is acknowledged as the founding father of multiple family therapy (Asen & Scholz, 2010). In 1951 he began bringing the families of patients with psychosis together in a group in order to help them understand what was happening with their family member who was unwell, what schizophrenia was, and what treatments were being used and why. Being with other families in a group seemed to help not only the relatives but also the patient. Over a period of 15 years, Laqueur was able to reduce readmissions to hospital by 80%.

Multiple family therapy is now used with a wide range of problems, including psychosis, schizophrenia, eating disorders, substance misuse, the management of pain and chronic illness, and child abuse and neglect. It is a systemic therapeutic approach, which in the UK owes much to the influence of the anti-psychiatry movement (Szasz, 1974) and to Minuchin's work on the effects of social context and poverty (Minuchin *et al*, 1967). It also connects back to the emergence of groupwork in the UK and the social-change ethos of the ragged schools movement (Webster, 1973). In the UK, multiple family therapy is epitomised by the work of Asen, Cooklin, Dawson, Eisler, McHugh; the Marlborough Family Service[7] in London (Asen *et al*, 2001; Asen & Scholz, 2010; Dawson & McHugh, 2012); and the eating disorders service at the Maudsley Hospital.

Asen and Scholz (2010) have a table that sets out their rationale for multi-family therapy. It contains many of the elements that have emerged from my own conversations with NVR participants and facilitators, but omits the particular value of having a diverse group. Their table includes:

- creating solidarity
- overcoming stigmatisation and social isolation
- stimulating new perspectives
- learning from each other
- being mirrored in others
- positive use of group pressure
- mutual support and feedback
- discovering and building on competencies
- experimenting with 'foster' families and swapping
- intensifying interactions and experiences
- raising hopes
- practising new behaviours in a safe space
- strengthening self-reflectiveness
- promoting openness and increasing self-confidence through 'public' exchanges and interactions.

Many of these elements are among the therapeutic factors identified by Yalom and Lesczc (2005) as influencing the process of change and recovery among clients

7 The Marlborough Family Service has sadly closed down. It had a 40-year history of doing multi-family work, and the model it developed is known as the Marlborough Family Model.

 

in all kinds of group therapy:

- Universality – a feeling of having problems similar to others, not being alone.
- Altruism – helping and supporting others.
- Instillation of hope – encouragement that recovery is possible.
- Guidance – nurturing support and assistance.
- Imparting information – teaching about problems and recovery.
- Developing social skills – learning new ways to talk about feelings, observations and concerns.
- Interpersonal learning – finding out about themselves and others from the group.
- Cohesion – feeling of belonging to the group, valuing the group.
- Catharsis – release of emotional tension.
- Existential factors – life and death are realities.
- Imitative behaviour – modelling another's manners and recovery skills.
- Corrective recapitulation of family of origin issues – identifying and changing the dysfunctional patterns or roles one played in one's primary family.

Therapeutic factors in NVR therapy:

- Identifying personal values and their origins (gender, culture, religion, family, upbringing) and fitting these into universal parenting values.
- Committing to non-violence (words, feelings and actions).
- Breaking the taboo of silence.
- Graduate parent participation.
- Persistence.
- Finding and promoting reconnection.
- Recognising relational patterns and committing to rebuilding positive patterns.
- Finding a sense of purpose and feeling grounded.
- Experiencing an embodied sense of parental presence.
- Learning and using mindfulness practices.
- Sharing experiences and hurts.
- Developing support networks.

- Envisioning and holding onto hope and love.
- Repositioning – getting a feel for the child's experience and trauma.
- Forgiveness – forgiving oneself and others and asking for forgiveness from others.
- Witnessing and supporting others.
- Experimenting with new ways of living and doing relationships.
- Laughing together.

I am struck by how NVR foregrounds values and beliefs. NVR is about what you do but also about what you believe and how you do things. Like multiple family therapy, it involves far more than teaching parents skills and techniques.

Multiple family therapy encourages entire families to be therapeutic with one another, while the therapist decentres herself (Asen & Scholz, 2010). Our programme does this with parents while focusing on how they can be therapeutic with their children.

Our intervention was developed by family therapists but is not family therapy in its traditional form. Somc of our parents will already have had family therapy, or will go on to have family therapy after the programme finishes, and this element is built in to the Latin American NVR project developed by Gilda Flores Acqueveque (Day & Flores Acqueveque, 2014). Our therapy programme was developed by systemic family therapists and uses a systemic approach as well as systemic methods and techniques (Burnham, 1992) and this locates it firmly within the systemic tradition.

Where hierarchies have become reversed in the home, parents are encouraged to take responsibility for making changes and responding in a different way, and the focus should be on them. So we do not see the group as one in which whole families come together but one in which the adults are the primary focus.

Multiple family therapy usually focuses on a specific presenting problem. Ivan Eisler and his team at the Maudsley hospital run a well-known and well-researched multiple family therapy group for young people with eating disorders (Eisler, 2005), which the whole family attends. At points during the sessions parents and children are seen separately, but it is essentially a programme for the entire family. A similar programme runs in Dresden in Germany. The purpose of these programmes is somewhat different from ours, as they are specifically focused on reducing the symptoms of anorexia nervosa through a programme of enactment (families eating meals together) and by supporting parents to develop skills and strategies to manage and endure the ensuing escalation and patterns of conflict (Eisler, 2005; Scholz *et al*, 2005). While our programme is ostensibly built around a common presenting problem, it is the particular combination of parents' distress and hopelessness coupled with cyclical patterns of escalation that invites non-violent resistance therapy as a clinical intervention.

I would argue strongly that NVR therapy is an inherently systemic way of working with parents, just as multiple family therapy is inherently systemic. NVR pays attention to the many stories in families, particularly those untold and unheard stories of strength and resilience (Pearce & Pearce, 1998). It values clients as important authors of these new stories and experts in 'local knowledge' (Geertz, 1983) – the ways in which their own families work. In the NVR therapy programme the involvement of graduate parents, and their specific role, acknowledges and harnesses this strength and expertise: parents reposition themselves in relation to the problem that first brought them to the group and become a resource and a story of hope for new parents.

An NVR approach may be indicated when the child's violent or self-destructive behaviour shows itself within a particular relational pattern: the parents have lost parental presence. In their interaction with their children, such parents frequently exhibit high levels of expressed emotion (Brown *et al*, 1972) – in their response to challenging behaviour they can be unnecessarily punitive or far too submissive. Incidents escalate quickly and end up in verbal or physical violence, or in parents giving in to their child's demands. Many parents find themselves alternating their responses: sometimes they end up screaming and shouting, at other times they give in. This leaves them feeling demoralised and ineffective.

# Research

In the UK and elsewhere there is much emphasis on measuring clinical outcomes. It is important to know if an intervention works, but measuring outcomes cannot tell us what is going on and how change happens. Evidence-based practice 'often relies on manualised approaches, thus silencing creativity in the therapeutic practice, marginalising relational inclinations, restricting therapists' capacity to respond to clients' unique circumstances' (Tilsen & McNamee, 2015). In this way of thinking about research there is a focus on adherence to the model or manual, which does not fit with an evolving intervention like NVR.

Self-report scales are seen as less reliable than other sorts of evidence because they are vulnerable to the halo effect (Nisbett & DeCamp Wilson, 1977) or social pressure to conform (Jupp, 2006; Northrup 1996). However, what people tell us about their experience is important and relevant.

Many organisations see randomised control trials (RCTs) as the gold standard in evidence-based research (Grossman & Mackenzie, 2005). A properly funded RCT involves teams of clinicians and researchers working for several years. Subjects are allocated randomly either to a specific treatment arm or to treatment as usual (TAU). An RCT scores highly in terms of traditional standards of validity, reliability and transferability. The self-harm intervention, family therapy (SHIFT) trial is a good example of a large, pragmatic intervention trial that has been undertaken over three sites (Leeds, Manchester, London). It has tested the effectiveness of a manualised family therapy intervention for young people with repeated self-harm. This study is the largest complex intervention trial yet undertaken in child mental health (Boston & Cottrell, 2016).

Non-violent resistance RCTs are under way in Holland and Germany. If funding were available, it would in principle be possible to set up an RCT in the UK that compares our manualised programme with treatment as usual. But there is no obvious treatment as usual for our families because of the complexity of their problems. To compare our programme with parenting programmes such as Webster-Stratton and Triple P would not be to compare like with like. RCTs depend on the intervention being provided in the same way each time.

Our NVR programme contains pre- and post- self-report measures designed to assess participants' levels of disturbance in three areas: distress, being out of control, and levels of support (Subjective Units of Disturbance Scale – SUDS). We have routinely used a number of other standard questionnaires to assess parents' levels of anxiety and depression and conflict in the family. In the past we have also had access to Strength and Difficulties Questionnaires (SDQ), Revised Children's Anxiety and Depression Scale (RCADS) and Children's Global Assessment Scale (CGAS) scores for the children and young people whose parents we were seeing.

However, because the programme is not included in the list of approved evidence-based interventions, it has sometimes been difficult to get support or even agreement to analyse the data collected. In one local authority, the NVR programme showed better outcomes than the other parenting interventions which the department was running, but this information was not included in reports because the NVR programme was not on the list of approved programmes. There may have also been funding issues for programmes not on the list.

The effectiveness of NVR is cited in The National Institute for Health and Care Excellence, Quality Standards and Indicators: Conduct Disorders (2013, p36), which is a step towards a more formal recognition of the programme.

> *'Non–violent resistance: a number of family and systemic psychotherapists … are developing ways of working with families affected by conduct disorders using non-violent resistance (NVR). An emerging evidence base for NVR demonstrates behavioural improvement in young people and in parents, an over 90% retention rate in therapy, reduced parental helplessness, improved parent mental health and improved perception of social support in parents compared to controls.'*

Each NVR group is unique: the growth and development of the participants is shaped in joint action. Participants create new stories together, and each group affects the way in which the next group is run. The process is living and dynamic and demands a research method that can capture that and do it justice.

Practice Based Evidence Based Practice PBEBP (van Hennick & Hillewaere, 2017) is an example of practitioner research. Participants and facilitators/ therapists become researchers and co-researchers together, in order to understand what they are creating and how to do it better. This is process research rather than outcome research (Burck & Simon, 2017).

# Conclusion

Haim Omer (2010) describes NVR as moving parents from speaking from an 'I' to a 'we' position. Such typically systemic repositioning reduces isolation and creates networks and systems of concern (Lang & McAdam, 1995). This firmly locates NVR in the field of therapeutic groupwork, where it owes more to the heritage of multiple family work than to the parenting group interventions that it superficially resembles.

Glynn *et al* (2006) and Price-Robertson (2017), quoted in Jewell and Lemmens (2018), observe that, 'the non-pathologising stance, the use of a collaborative approach, the inclusion of mutual self-help and peer support in MFT (multiple family therapy) makes it consistent with a relational approach to recovery that has family life at its heart'.

Hubble *et al* (1999) remind us that that what really counts in successful therapy is the therapeutic alliance, the therapist's allegiance to their clients and their expectation of change. The NVR programme builds in these elements and also incorporates tangible self-actualisation (Maslow, 1943).

The methods of NVR (announcements, sit-ins, reconciliation gestures) are performative (Butler, 1997). They are performances of active resistance in the face of violence and oppression. They seek to bring about positive change in a radical (non-traditional and non-mainstream) way, because that is the ethical thing to do. Each time parents and facilitators perform the principles of NVR they carry out an embodied performance (Denzin, 2003; 2006) that communicates at a range of levels from the educational to the inspirational to the transformational.

## References

Appleton R, Douglas H & Rheeston M (2016) Taking part in 'Understanding Your Child's Behaviour' and positive changes for parents. *Community Practitioner* **89** 2 42–48.

Asen E, Dawson N & McHugh B (2001) *Multiple Family Therapy: The Marlborough Model and its wider applications*. London: Karnac.

Asen E & Scholz M (2010) *Multi-Family Therapy: Concepts and techniques*. London: Routledge.

Bateson G (1973) *Steps to an Ecology of Mind.* London: Paladin.

Bateson G (1979) *Mind and Nature.* New York: Dutton.

Bion WR (1961) *Experiences in Groups*. New York: Basic Books.

Boston P & Cottrell D (2016) Trials and Tribulations – an RCT comparing manualized family therapy with Treatment as Usual and reflections on key issues that arose in the implementation. *Journal of Family Therapy* pp172–188.

Brown GW, Birley JL & Wing JK (1972) Influence of family life on the course of schizophrenic disorders: a replication. *British Journal of Psychiatry* **121** pp241–258.

Burck C & Simon G (2017) Developments in systemic practitioner research. *Journal of Family Therapy* **39** pp285–287.

Burnham J (1992) Approach–method–technique: making distinctions and creating connections. *Human Systems* **3** pp3–27.

Burr V (1995) *An Introduction to Social Constructionism*. London: Routledge.

Butler J (1997) *Excitable Speech: A politics of the performative*. New York: Routledge.

Dawson N & McHugh B (2012) The history and development of Marlborough multi-family groups in education. *Context*, **123**, pp 8-11.

Day C, Michelson D, Thomson S, Penney C & Draper L (2012a) Evaluation of a peer-led parenting intervention for disruptive behaviour problems in children: community based randomised controlled trial. *British Medical Journal* **344** pe1107.

Day C, Michelson D, Thomson S, Penney C & Draper L (2012b) Innovations in practice: empowering parents, empowering communities: a pilot evaluation of a peer-led parenting programme. *Child and Adolescent Mental Health* **17** (1) 52–57.

Day EM & Flores Acqueveque G (2014) Non-violent resistance: a community-group programme for Latin American families. *Context* **132** pp32–33.

Day EM & Heismann E (2010) *Non-violent Resistance Programme*. Hove: Pavilion Publishing.

Department for Education (2015) 2010 to 2015 government policy: looked-after children and adoption [online]. Available at: www.education.gov.uk/childrenandyoungpeople/families/childrenincare/news/a0075693/prospectus (accessed November 2018).

 

Denzin NK (2003) *Performance Ethnography: Critical pedagogy and the politics of culture*. London: Sage.

Denzin NK (2006) *The politics and ethics of performance pedagogy: Toward a pedagogy of hope*. In: DS Madison & J Hamera (eds) *The Sage Handbook of Performance Studies*. Thousand Oaks, CA: Sage.

Eisler I (2005) The empirical and theoretical base of family therapy and multiple family day therapy for adolescent anorexia nervosa. *Journal of Family Therapy* **27**(2) pp104–131.

Furman R, Rowan D & Bender K (2009) *An Experiential Approach to Group Work*. Chicago: Lyceum Books.

Geertz C (1983) *Local Knowledge*. New York: Basic Books.

Gergen KJ (2001) *Social Construction in Context*. London: Sage.

Gergen KJ (2009) *An Invitation to Social Constructionism*. Second Edition. London: Sage.

Grossman J & Mackenzie FJ (2005) The randomized controlled trial: gold standard, or merely standard? *Perspectives in Biology and Medicine* **48**(4) pp516–34.

Hayden C & Molenkamp RJ (2002) *The Tavistock Primer II* [online]. AK Rice Institute for the Study of Social Systems. Available at: https://nycgrouprelations.org/wp-content/uploads/2018/06/AKRITavistockPrimerII.pdf (accessed November 2018).

Hubble M, Duncan B & Miller S (1999) *The Heart and Soul of Change*. Washington DC: APA.

Jewell T & Lemmens G (2018) Multiple Family Therapy: Forever promising? Commentary on Gelin et al (2018) and Cook-Darzens et al (2018) The evidence base for Multiple Family Therapy in psychiatric and non-psychiatric conditions: a review (parts 1 and 2). *Journal of Family Therapy* **40** pp344–348.

Jupp V (2006) *The Sage Dictionary of Social Research Methods*. Sage.

Kurland R & Salmon R (1993) Not just one of the gang: group workers and their role as an authority. *Social Work with Groups: A journal of community and clinical practice* **16**(1-2) 153–169.

Laqueur HP (1972) *Mechanics of change in multiple family therapy*. In: CJ Sager & HS Kaplan (Eds) *Progress in Group and Family Therapy*. New York: Bruner/Mazel.

Lang P & McAdam E (1995) Referrals, referrers and the system of concern. *Human Systems* **6** pp71–103.

Macbeth A, Law J, Mcgowan I, Norrie J, Thompson L & Wilson P (2015) Mellow parenting: systematic review and meta-analysis of an intervention to promote sensitive parenting. *Developmental Medicine & Child Neurology*.

Maslow AH (1943) A Theory of Human Motivation. *Psychological Review* **50** pp370–396.

Maturana HR & Varela FJ (1980) *Autopoiesis and Cognition: The Realization of the Living*. Dordrecht: Holland.

McNamee S & Gergen KJ (1992) *Therapy as Social Construction*. London: Sage.

Minuchin S, Montalvo B, Guerney G, Rosman B & Schumer F (1967) *Families of the Slums: An exploration of their structure and treatment*. New York: Basic Books.

Montgomery (2002) Role of dynamic group therapy in psychiatry. *Advances in Psychiatric Treatment* **8** pp34–41.

National Institute for Health and Care Excellence (2013) *Quality Standards and Indicators Briefing Paper: Conduct Disorders*.

Nisbett RE & DeCamp Wilson T (1977) The Halo effect: evidence for unconscious alteration of judgments. *Journal of Personality and Social Psychology* **35** (4) pp250–256.

Northrup DA (1996) The problem of the self-report in survey research. *Institute of Social Research Newsletter*. **11** (3).

Omer H (2010) *The New Authority*. Cambridge: Cambridge University Press.

Pearce WB & Pearce KA (1998) Transcendent storytelling: abilities for systemic practitioners and their clients. *Human Systems* **9** pp167–185.

Pratt JH (1905) The class method of treating consumption in the homes of the poor. In: KR MacKensie (ed) (1992) *Classics in Group Psychotherapy*. New York: Guildford Press.

Preston-Shoot M (2007) *Effective Groupwork*. Basingstoke: Palgrave Macmillan.

Scholz M, Rix M, Scholz K, Gantchev K & Thömke V (2005) Multiple family therapy for anorexia nervosa: concepts, experiences and results. *Journal of Family Therapy* **27** (2) pp132–141.

Shotter J (2012) More than cool reason: 'withness-thinking' or 'systemic thinking' and 'thinking about systems'. *International Journal of Collaborative Practices* **3** (1) pp1–13.

Shotter J (2016) *Speaking, Actually: Towards a new 'fluid' common-sense understanding of relational becomings*. Farnhill: Everything is Connected Press.

Smith MK (2004) *The early development of group work* [online]. Available at: www.infed.org/groupwork/early_group_work.htm (accessed October 2018).

Steele M, Marigna M, Tello J & Johnson R (2000) *Strengthening Families, Strengthening Communities: An inclusive parent programme*. London: Race Equality Foundation.

Szasz T (1974) *The Myth of Mental Illness*. New York: Harper Row.

The New York Center for the Study of Groups, Organizations, and Social Systems. (2014) *Tavistock Model* [online]. Available at: http://www.nycgrouprelations.org/pdf/TavistockModel.pdf

Thomson RM, Allely CS, Purves D, Puckering C, McConnachie A, Johnson PCD, Golding J, Gillberg C & Wilson P (2014) Predictors of positive and negative parenting behaviours: evidence from the ALSPAC cohort. *BMC Pediatrics* **14** 247.

Tilsen J & McNamee S (2015) Feedback informed treatment: Evidence-based practice meets social construction. *Family Process* **54** pp124–137.

van Hennick R & Hillewaere B (2017) Practice Based Evidence Based Practice. Navigating based on coordinated improvisation, collaborative learning and multi-methods research in Feedback Informed Systemic Therapy. *Journal of Family Therapy* **39** pp288–309.

Webster DH (1973) *The Ragged School Movement and the Education of the Poor in the Nineteenth Century.* Unpublished Doctoral Thesis. University of Leicester.

Webster-Stratton C (2009) *Overview of the Webster-Stratton parent training programme.* For more information, see www.incredibleyears.com (accessed October 2018).

Webster-Stratton C, Reid JM & Beauchaine TP (2013) One-Year Follow-Up of Combined Parent and Child Intervention for Young Children with ADHD. *Journal of Clinical Child & Adolescent Psychology* **42** (2) pp251–261.

Wittgenstein L (1953) *Philosophical Investigations.* Oxford: Blackwell.

Yalom ID & Lesczc M (2005) *The Theory and Practice of Group Psychotherapy*. New York, NY: Basic Books.

 

# Chapter 16: 'Statistics are needed for the professionals to keep running the course, but it is living proof that keeps the parents attending'

**By Elisabeth Heismann**

## Introduction

Over the past ten years, the input of graduate parents has become a central force in the evolution of my own approach to NVR practice and training. Graduate parent participation is also steadily becoming more mainstream within many UK-based NVR practices. The participatory aspect of NVR group interventions makes the approach particularly effective, even with people who have been difficult to reach or have experienced resistance to other interventions. The development of participatory work with graduate parents in NVR has close links with other participatory practices and practical influences, which underpin the concepts of the participatory approach in NVR group work. This chapter looks at the contributions made by Paulo Freire, Michael White and David Epston in relation to graduate parent work in NVR.

I start with Paulo Freire, who developed participatory practice in the early 70s in the field of adult education. I then look at Michael White's ground-breaking discourses on participatory narrative practice and the influences of David

Epston's performative processes in narrative-based work. I use these stepping stones to reflect on the relevance of the participatory process, when involving graduate parents in NVR work. My aim is to encourage other practitioners to continue developing NVR as participatory practice by expanding the discourse around theoretical influences on NVR parent work.

## Participatory education

The idea of participation and collaboration as functions of the education process entered my life in the 1970s when I was transitioning into teaching in Germany. During this time, I also became a member of a social activist group that was supporting a co-operative of Portuguese farm labourers. 'Soldado Luis' had formed following the 'Revolution of the Carnations' in 1974 and, as a result of the 'land reform', land had been allocated to them which had previously belonged to the Patron. By the time of our involvement, the co-operative's members had started to decide upon and run their own affairs. We helped them farm the cork trees, worked with them in the rice fields, and also contributed financially to their cause.

In 1980, a two-year alphabetisation[8] campaign for adults started in the local area. This work was based on the participatory concepts of learning that were developed by the Brazilian educator Paulo Freire. They had been initially tried out in Latin America and were later adopted throughout the developing world. Freire's approach to literacy was revolutionary as it joined the process of '*reading the word*' with '*reading the world*' (Freire, 1987, p182). Freire called it the 'dialogical active participation method' in his book *Pedagogy of the Oppressed* (Freire, 1972) as it requires a dialogical exchange between teachers and students, where both learn, both question, both reflect and both participate in meaning-making. The teacher uses the real-life situations of the learners as the starting point for a shared investigative journey that takes place between teachers and learners.

The aim of this method is to help people develop critical consciousness through critical thinking styles, thus finding new approaches to overcoming obstacles that have kept them from moving forward. The process of developing literacy begins with the teachers as investigators, immersing themselves in the communities they want to work with. Their task at this stage is for the teachers, supported by co-investigators (members within the learner group), to collect and develop a list of 'generative words and themes' (Freire 1972, p69) (generative words are words that are relevant to the daily lives of the people). These 'generative words and

8 According to Freire, education starts with literacy, learning the spelling of relevant words that are shared by the community of learners, thereby developing a growing awareness of yourself and your social world. Naming the world is a step towards *conscientisation*.

 

themes' are 'coded' into materials (pictures, texts, films, drama) that will enable the participants to 'decode', understand, critically examine and reflect on their social reality, starting the process of 'conscientisation'. 'Conscientisation' allows, *'reflection and action upon the world in order to transform it'* (Freire, 1972, p24–28)

Through critical reflection in dialogue and co-operation with the teacher and each other, they start acting on this reality and transform it. This enables them to move from being 'objects' to 'subjects', giving them agency in their own lives. This is referred to as 'authentic praxis' as it emerges directly from participants' experiences. Their narratives are communicated, reflected on and acted on. Reflection then expands to a shared process of 'reflection in action'. Participation in the struggle for liberation leads to the development of a stance of 'committed involvement' among both teachers and participants (Freire, 1972, p44). The narratives provide a thread between past, present and future, and serve to free up new possibilities.

> *'Looking at the past must only be a means of understanding more clearly what and who they are so that they can more wisely build the future. They emerge from their 'here and now' situation and start to "intervene" in their reality, as they perceive their situation no longer as "limiting" but as "challenging"'* (Freire, 1972, pp57–63).

Seeing the situation as a challenge allows people to externalise the problem and move away from feeling helpless and hopeless. This dialogical encounter is based on 'love', 'humility', 'faith', 'mutual trust' and 'hope' between teachers and learners leading to non-judgemental 'critical thinking' (Freire, 1972, p65). By externalising their important themes, participants are able to perceive their viewpoints as 'perceptions', enabling them to develop new knowledge about self and the ability to experiment with different perceptions and actions, which Freire calls 'testing actions'.

'Testing actions' are used to negotiate the space between the previously perceived and unperceived obstacles and solutions (Freire, 1972, p95). The dialogical encounter is mutually beneficial. Teachers are *'authenticated in their praxis with the praxis of the people (thinking) with the people, not for the people'* (Freire, 1972, pp100–101). It is essential that teachers approach this process with humility, that they are not prescriptive, self-interested or analytical of the learners, which would be another form of 'domination' and 'cultural invasion' (Freire, 1972, pp122–139). The processes of 'witnessing' enables all the participants, including the teachers and the learners, to become 'co-authors' of the learning and living process, leading to the 'enrichment of both' (Freire, 1972, pp144–48).

In our participatory NVR groups, new participants immediately connect with parent facilitators, who share their own lived experiences, similar to those that the new parents are still going through, thereby enabling dialogue and reflection in and on action right from the start. When sharing about having been in similar places themselves in the past, but now feeling at a different stage in their testimonies and dialogues, parent facilitators are thinking *with* new parent participants with empathy, humility and compassion, and not *for* them, while always foregrounding the new parents' current relevant themes and difficulties. In the following section I will look at Michael White's ideas on participation in the therapeutic context.

## 'Externalising-the-problem', 'storying experience' and 're-authoring lives': Michael White's contribution to participatory praxis in therapy

During the early 1990s, while training to be a family therapist in London, I was introduced to the innovative approach of the 'reflecting team', which was initially conceived by Tom Andersen and expanded by the Australian writer and therapist Michael White. The 'reflecting team' approach and White's concepts of 'externalising' and 're-authoring' felt like a natural progression from my previous experience of participation and collaborative processes in the co-operative and in the classroom. White describes the approach of 'externalising', where clients are encouraged to 'objectify and, at times, to personify the problems that they experience as oppressive. In this process, the problem becomes a separate entity and thus external to the person or relationship that was ascribed as the problem' (White & Epston, 1990, p38). This process allows that previously perceived inherent or fixed qualities become 'less fixed and less restricting' (White & Epston, 1990, ibid).

The 'problem-saturated descriptions' of life or the 'dominant stories' have led to stuckness, blaming and failure. Externalising makes space for 'alternative stories', for co-operation with others and taking action. Thus clients 'retrieve their lives and relationships from the problem and its influence' (White, 1990, p39). Here the focus is on the person's relationship with the problem rather than on the problem itself (White & Epston, 1990, p40). Although the dominant stories shape people's lives, they *'do not sufficiently represent their lived experience …(because the 'unique outcomes' which are frequently left out in the re-telling) contradict these dominant narratives'* (White & Epston, 1990, p41). These 'unique outcomes' can be plotted together to form alternative stories.

This process leads to the 're-authoring of lives and relationships' (White & Epston, 1990, ibid). This approach is particularly useful when dealing with experiences and stories of violence and abuse, where attitudes and beliefs, rather than the violence itself, are 'externalised' (White & Epston, 1990, p49). 'Externalising' can also offer people with conflicting perspectives the opportunity to 'establish a mutually acceptable definition of the problem and facilitate conditions under which persons can work together to resolve their problems' (White & Epston 1990, p54). Drawing from his work with families, White proposes that it is helpful but not necessary for those who have a relationship with the problem to be actively engaged in generating and performing new meanings (White & Epston 1990, p59). He says that, *'it is never the size of the step that a person takes that counts but its direction'*, and that 'unique outcomes' sometimes present themselves in the course of the session or afterwards and that it is the therapist's role to be receptive to any 'news of difference' (White & Epston, 1990, ibid) while the client's role is to start taking responsibility for the problem and *'refuse(s) to co-operate with the requirements of the problem,* [thereby] *undermining it...* [allowing them to foster a] *'new sense of personal agency …* [giving them the tools] *to intervene in their world'* (White & Epston, 1990, pp61–65).

White positions this therapeutic process as a 'counter-practice' to the culture of objectification allowing the process of 're-authoring' through alternative stories, new knowledge and subjectivity (White & Epston 1990, p75). In NVR, the concept of connection before correction enables parents to separate the child from the problem. They develop the ability to make meaningful connections with their child, even when things are difficult, and learn to appreciate connection as more important than correction. An important step is helping them to prioritise or externalise their long list of problems in the work with different-sized baskets using their core parenting values.

In the following section, I will describe how David Epston developed the concept of 'Insider Witnessing Practice' as a counterpoint practice to White's approach.

## 'Insider Witnessing Practice' as a performance-based narrative approach

David Epston worked closely with White for many years. He developed his concept of 'Insider Witnessing Practice' (IWP) after White's death as a counterpoint to the 'Outsider Witness Practices' (OWP). While in OWP strangers convey regard and respect, in IWP an 'intimate other' not only re-stories but 'performs' the narrative, capturing the 'essence', 'qualities of character' and 'history' (Carlson, 2017, Part Two, p21). The narrative process in art and in therapy allows someone to be simultaneously 'author' and 'character' in their own story, sensing themselves in the process of acting and making (Carlson, 2017, Part Two, p24). Through performance, an 'audience' emerges and through 'witnessing' they are 'brought to tears, become angry and called to some response' (Carlson, 2017, Part Two, ibid).

Intimacy develops in the audience, author, and character relationships where the client witnesses the performance of their own story as 'not me, but not not me' (Carlson, 2017, Part Two, p25). Epston's IWPs comprises of two acts: in the first act the 'portraying therapist' (PT) is interviewed by another narrative therapist or supervisor as if they were the client, extending the story beyond the 'so-far-known' and including a 'hope-biased counter-history' (Carlson, 2017, Part Two, p27). In the second act, the client or 'person portrayed' (PP), becomes a witness to the 'portraying therapist's' performance that was developed in the first act, thereby becoming 'both an insider and an outsider to her own story… [allowing her] to feel and experience levels of self-endearment and self-love that are usually reserved only for respected others … Mutuality of respect is given abundant expression by the therapist's portrayal and in return, the portrayed person reciprocates by doing something similar for themselves' (Carlson, 2017, Part Two, p28–33).

The witnessing in NVR happens through parent facilitators' testimonies being performed live in front of new parents, where often feelings are expressed in great depth or where sometimes the audience breaks out in laughter in recognition of the similarity of the stories told and lived. In graduation ceremonies, to which guests, supporters and public figures like borough police commissioners are invited, some parents do not feel ready to read out their own testimonies but ask someone else to read them on their behalf. These experiences link with what Epston calls being inside a witness, where you see, feel and hear their testimony.

In the following section, I will explore how the ideas of participation are relevant for working with graduate parents in NVR.

## Graduate parent participation in NVR group work

In 2006 I came across the ideas and practices of NVR through a training session with Haim Omer while working in a London Child and Adolescent Mental Health Service (CAMHS). My colleagues and I were immediately drawn to the approach as the ideas directly applied to the families and situations we were working with. The first pilot group was launched in 2007. The participation of parents who had 'graduated' (having attended at least five weeks of the programme) was a natural progression for us during the third programme. The regular participation of 'graduate parents' subsequently became the most unique and important feature of our parent groups, inspiring professionals and prospective parents as well as re-inspiring the graduate parents themselves. Within the last 10 years, 'graduate parent' participation has become mainstream in a lot of NVR group work in the UK.

The graduate parents demonstrate and embody the aspects of NVR that facilitate sustainable positive change, which are the level of 'parental presence', 'support', and 'protective action' and the four parental values ('safety', 'developing the child's potential and abilities', 'staying connected and enjoying a good relationship with each other' and 'showing respect for themselves and for others' (Grabbe, 2013, p71). Graduate parent testimonies enable new parents to access these concepts more openly and reframe their critical, defensive, helpless and hopeless perceptions towards a willingness to learn new skills. Graduate parents help participants with the challenges of negotiating the dynamics with the professionals, other group members and the NVR process itself. Being witness to graduate parents who have been able to overcome similar limitations as themselves, allows for participants to go through the process of 'conscientisation', becoming 'experimental' (Dewey, 1938, p79) with interventions into their own realities, using 'testing actions', which can be supported and critically reflected upon afterwards.

Receiving the commitment, humility, wisdom, support, solidarity, hope and love of everyone involved, including facilitators, and experiencing everyone as supporters and equals, cultivates a shared 'quest for information and for production of new ideas' (Dewey, 1938, p79), giving rise to further experiences in which new problems present themselves. This experimental method is a 'continual spiral' (Dewey, 1938, ibid). Graduate parents' participation contributes to the joint dialogical investigation that the group undertakes, where the sharing of 'lived', 'told', 'untellable', and 'unheard' stories (Pearce, 2007, p212) leads to the 'continuous formations' and 'readjustments of selves' (Dewey, 2011, p191) in the process of 'self-actualisation' (Maslow, 2012) and the development of the 'art of loving' (Fromm, 1957) and 'human completion' (Freire, 1970, p24).

The physical presence and spiritual guidance of the graduate parents have an 'anchor function' (Omer, 2011) for the participants. Their support does not replace the role of the professional facilitators or other professionals but expands their 'anchoring function' as graduate parent input is more organic, familiar and accessible than the professionals, even though facilitators often refer to their own parenting experiences in relation to NVR to connect more authentically with participants. The presence of graduate parents offers facilitators another layer of witnessing, which enables them to reflect on and act into their own narratives and approach.

The support function of the graduate parents for others and to each other seems to be the most obvious aspect that parents have identified in interviews, questionnaires or in conversations, exemplified in statements like the following:

*'I have gained more support from like-minded people who understand what it is I am trying to achieve.'*

*'Just everyone is there to support each other.'*

*'Making a stand helps other people make that stand.'*

*'One person can't change things on their own.'*

*'Supporters are vital to NVR.'*

*'They'll help other parents and they'll help themselves.'*

*'We are supporters, aren't we, to the programme.'*

*'We are there to support each other.'*

The graduate parents feel their involvement with new parent groups helps them stay persistent with their own families. Graduate parents embody what we try to convey in our teaching of the key principles: I am not alone. If necessary I can draw on social support. Isolated parents have often imprisoned themselves in order to hide feelings of guilt and shame (Weinblatt, 2016) and initially find it difficult to name any support for themselves or their child. In the safe environment of the group, where they experience solidarity, empathy and understanding instead of the prejudice and judgement that they expect from others, they often learn to trust again or sometimes to trust others for the first time. Professionals often too quickly turn to solutions when they are facing these situations, while graduate parents can more easily identify and empathise with this position of loneliness and low mood as shown in the following quotes:

*'I know exactly how they are feeling, how low they feel.'*

*'I have been stood in your shoes.'*

*'I thought it was just us and everybody else's family was perfect'*

*'You can see people begin to understand things more if they speak to somebody who has been actually through it. I can't imagine it without it. It's really an important part of NVR to me.'*

*'NVR is effective having graduate parents actively involved during the parent groups, as they are the voice that tells the reality of how the NVR tools were used to achieve positive changes with their child's challenging behaviour. Parents relate to this as our stories are real, not from a book.'*

The question is: what is there to learn from all the presented historical and current participatory approaches in a contemporary context, where knowledge and resources are banked and accumulated in the hands of few? Freire guided us away from this exclusive banking approach in adult education and enabled teachers and learners to communicate and dialogue at eye-level and inclusively. There can be challenges and pitfalls, as our NVR parent facilitators and professional facilitators regularly alert us about: parent facilitators can be overused or overexposed, and their enthusiasm to give something back can put them at risk, for example when they venture into other parent's homes on their own or when unfamiliar with organisational protocols or safeguarding procedures. In those circumstances expert knowledge can guide them.

However, we see them at all times as the experts on their own stories and lived experiences, but not on those of others. Externalising problem behaviours and unhelpful, harmful patterns of relating to others and witnessing the experience of others and selves, hearing, feeling and seeing them through performance and enactments have always been our preferred ways of collaborating with parents, guided by the ideas and practices of Michael White, David Epston and others like Augusto Boals' work in theatre (Boal, 2000). We believe that people not only participate in speech between each other, but our own and other people's bodies and feelings need to be equally mindfully integrated as speech in all aspects of our work for a fully participatory NVR approach.

## Concluding thoughts

As has become evident, these social cultural and conceptual developments have greatly influenced my own thinking and therapeutic and community-based practices, and have directly led me to my conviction in the reciprocal benefits of participatory work with graduate parents in NVR. This chapter has looked at the participatory approach of NVR group interventions as one of the most important parts of the NVR group programme. In our experience of NVR work, graduate parents have enabled us to be particularly effective in recruiting and retaining parents who were reluctant to come in the first place or who did not plan to stay, many of whom have become active and passionate advocates of the approach and are actively involved in the programmes.

The development of this participatory practice has a valuable contribution to make to the discourses around participation in community and therapeutic practice. A greater awareness of the historical roots of participatory practice helps us to think about how relevant participatory practice remains today for social and for self-development. The work with graduate parents in NVR could lead the way forward in this respect.

It is my hope that practitioners of the NVR approach continue collaborating with graduate parents and regard parent participation as a core aspect of their practice.

My heartfelt thanks go to all those graduate parents who have explicitly and implicitly contributed to this chapter.

## References

Andersen T (1990) *Das Reflektierende Team: Dialoge über die Dialoge*. Dortmund: Modernes Lernen.

Andersen T (1993) *The Reflecting Team: Dialogues and dialogues about dialogues*. Norton and Co.

Boal A (2000) *Theatre of the Oppressed*. London: Pluto Press.

Carlson TS & Epston D (2017). Insider Witnessing Practices: Part Two. *Journal of Narrative Family Therapy Release* **1** pp19–38.

Dewey J (1938, Free Press edition 2015) *Experience & Education*. The Kappa Delta Pi Lecture Series, Free Press New York.

Dewey J (2011) *Democracy and Education*, Milton Keynes.

Epston D (2016) The Corner. Re-imagining Narrative Therapy: A history for the future. *Journal of Systemic Therapies* **35** (1) pp79-87.

Freire P (1972) *Pedagogy of the Oppressed*. St Ives: Clays Ltd.

Freire P (1974, re-published 2013) *Education for Critical Consciousness*. London: Bloomsbury.

Freire P (1987) *A Pedagogy For Liberation. Dialogues on transforming education.* New York.

Fromm E (1957 Thorsons Edition 1995) St Ives: Clays Ltd,

Grabbe M (2013) *Wo fahren wir hin und wo ankern wir? Vom Navigieren in der Eltern-Kind -Beziehung*, chapter 3, pp 61-84. In: M Grabbe, J Borke, C Tsirigotis (HG) Autoritaet, Autonomie und Bindung. Die Ankerfunktion bei elterrlicher und professioneller Praesenz, Goettingen: Vandenhoeck & Ruprecht.

Maslow AH (2012) *Toward a Psychology of Being.* Start Publishing LAC 2012, USA.

Omer H (2011) *The New Authority. Family, school and community. New York: Cambridge* University Press.

Pearce BW (2007) *Making Social Worlds. A communication perspective*. Oxford: Blackwell Publishing Ltd.

Weinblatt U (2016) *Die Naehe ist ganz nah! Scham und Verletzungen in Beziehung ueberwinden,* Goettingen: Vandenhoeck & Ruprecht.

White M (1989) *Selected Papers*. Adelaide: Dulwich Centre Publications.

White M & Epston D (1990) *Narrative Means to Therapeutic Ends.* Adelaide: Dulwich Centre.

 

# Chapter 17: A group conversation about parent participation

22nd December 2017

## Key

New parent *
Parent facilitator #
Established parent facilitator ^
Professional facilitator ~

## Group members

| | |
|---|---|
| Elisabeth Heismann: | Moderator of the conversation and Professional Facilitator |
| Dorota Rospierska: | Professional Facilitator |
| Jacqui Swaden: | Established Parent Facilitator |
| Pete Brown: | Professional Facilitator |
| Jeanine Heismann: | Professional Facilitator |
| Lesley Wyvil: | Established Parent Facilitator |
| Carly Savage: | New Parent |
| Sukaena Cally: | Parent Facilitator |
| Angelique Smith: | Established Parent Facilitator |
| Linda Cakebread: | Established Parent Facilitator |
| Sarah Blyth: | Established Parent Facilitator |
| Chinyere Ikpala: | New Parent |
| Karina Kelly: | Parent Facilitator |
| Deborah Frimpong: | Established Parent Facilitator |
| Allison Rensch: | New Parent |
| Jane Prescott: | Professional Facilitator |
| Janet Akortsu: | New Parent |
| Ashley Farrugia: | New Parent |

**~Elisabeth: If you were asked to come up with a motto to describe parent participation as a core principle of our way of doing NVR, what would it be?**

~**Pete:** The glue that binds NVR together.

#**Karina:** Perfect balance, that complement each other, parents and professionals.

^**Linda:** It makes it real for parents rather than just hearing from professionals, who may have just learnt from books.

^**Angelique:** We are inspiring to anybody that participates.

^**Deborah:** I think people are learning through our experience. Learning through experience. Because our lifestyle or life experiences really make a big difference. Because each of us has a different life story.

~**Jeanine:** It also helps to bridge the gap.

*__Ashley:__ Parent action in NVR.

~**Pete:** Parent facilitators keep parents coming to the group.

**~Elisabeth: Have you been to parenting groups other than NVR? How would you describe the difference?**

^**Sarah:** I've been to one before. It had no parent facilitators, and it didn't really do much for me. It was more like parents sitting there just discussing the problems that are going on indoors. We had no parent facilitators there.

^**Lesley:** If you've got just the professionals there, it come across as if they are telling you what to do. They're the professionals, whereas when the parents are there, they're not just telling you of their successes and saying, '*There you are, you should do it like this. You should do it like that*'. They will also say, when things have not gone well, and how they have coped, and how they have not coped. And I think it makes it more real, because you understand that it is not always going to work. And how to adapt it for each individual family. If it's just professionals, they're just telling you, '*In this situation, you do it like this. In that situation, you do it like that*'. But it doesn't work. The parents tell you when it does, when it doesn't. What they've done, what they've not done and how they wished it had gone better.

~**Pete:** It makes it real.

 

**^Lesley:** Yes, and practical. A professional telling you what to do doesn't mean you are going to do what they say. You've got all that resistance, while when you hear, '*I have tried it. I have done it. It works*', you're perhaps less defensive.

**^Deborah:** With the parent facilitators there you get the empathy and compassion. Everybody's story is different. I came thinking: '*It is me*'. But then when I heard other people, I thought: '*Gosh, mine isn't that bad*'. I still thought it was difficult, but I thought: '*Somebody else is going through worse than me*'. So, I could have a different outlook on my situation and have compassion each week, when I came to hear other people's stories.

**^Lesley:** There is also someone there to break the ice to start with. If you're all going to sit there and say what your problems are, I think I would be very reluctant to open my mouth and I'd think, '*I don't want to tell all these people my problems*'. If a graduate parent tells you how difficult it has been and how they have moved on, you think, '*Maybe my issues are not so bad. Maybe, I could open my mouth and join in.*' So, I think it helps to break the ice quicker, because there is already somebody there who's prepared to open their mouth and tell their story.

**~Pete:** I run both NVR parenting groups and other parenting groups, where graduate parent facilitators aren't present. I think parenting groups without parent facilitators still have their value if the parents can be mobilised to talk about issues. But it doesn't have the same equal atmosphere. But the biggest thing for me is the dropout rate. With standard parenting groups, the dropout rate is extremely high. With NVR groups, it's very low.

**~Elisabeth: A teacher for adult literacy learning Paulo Freire called the participation approach '*authentic praxis*', where professionals work with learners in 'dialogue', which he describes as 'reflection on and in action', leading to knowing oneself and others and to choosing wise actions.**

**^Angelique:** From a parent's point of view, whatever you're speaking about is reality. And they feel it. In most of our cases and with our challenging circumstances, we have a lot of emotion about what we are going through. So straight away, that is, what others would see, especially as a new person, who is going through trauma. They just want to know that there are people who they can connect with, who are actually hearing them. You get a feeling of what they are feeling.

**~Dorota:** Parent facilitators are in a different emotional place and a different place of knowing themselves, and serve as a very positive example of taking responsibility, as opposed to feeling guilty for whatever the situation is. They speak with the other parents who come from a position that their child has to be fixed and ask them, '*What can you do? What kind of parent do you need to become for your child, to be able to make a positive change?*' The change in mindset is happening through the graduate parents' example, because it is implicit in those parents who are saying, 'I've changed my ways, and it helped my child to follow'. For me, it is about knowing oneself. But you can only do it after you have gone through a journey and have arrived in a different place from parents who are new and still in this very painful place and in the middle of a very difficult time.

**^Lesley:** That is, where you can help to move things along so much quicker. Because you can say, '*I was in that position. I came, because I had a difficult child. But this is what I am doing differently, and this is the result.*' So, I think it helps people to see that it is the way you are behaving towards your child and the way you are behaving in general at home which can change.

**^Deborah:** Yes, it's a conscious decision that you have to make. It's not just the child who's the problem. You're part of the equation, and that's the reality. When you get there, you're thinking, '*Why am I having to do this course? She is the problem. She is the one running away.*' And coming to that acceptance, that it is not just about your child, but that what you've been doing has caused an effect on the child. It's mind-blowing. And then being able to have somebody work with you through that. I remember a young lady – it wasn't when she was talking about all the wrong things that she was doing. It was when she was remembering the good things: '*My daughter was a good girl*'. That was when she broke down and started crying. She went to a place that she had completely forgotten. We think, '*I hate my child. I don't want to have anything to do with them*'. And then NVR helps you to reconnect to that place, where they're a baby, where they're helpless. And you just want to look after them. And then you just reconnect back to their childhood. So, I have got to do everything I can again.

**Do concepts like 'dialogue', 'self-knowledge', 'wise action' and 'reflection in and on action' make sense to you? If yes, do they fit with a moment in your experience with NVR, when you thought, 'Oh, that's it?'**

**^Deborah:** Yes, absolutely. Initially, you're trying to fix your child. And then you find out that you need to fix yourself; that you're broken. You're a broken person. And because you're a broken person, you were making some choices in your life that were having an effect on your child that were negative and producing this negative effect.

**^Lesley:** I didn't feel that I was broken or that I was doing something wrong. I thought, '*I'm not broken. It's not me who is doing everything wrong. I'm doing some things right, and nobody is judging me for the things that I'm not doing quite* *right for that child. It may have been fine for my other children, but it's not quite right for this one.*' So I actually felt much more empowered, thinking, '*I'm not such a bad parent after all*'.

**^Deborah:** I needed to find myself. I needed to find my brokenness to be able to deal with the situation that I had in hand. When I was writing things down in my self-announcement saying, '*My daughter is like this*', Elisabeth said, '*Try to write it differently*'. And I had to sit back thinking, '*I have a role in this*'. Whereas, when I first came, it was all her. Everything was her fault. And getting to that place where I asked myself, '*Where did you have any involvement?*' And then having to hold your hand and say, '*Don't feel guilty! You're doing it for the right reasons, but you were doing the wrong things*'. Arriving at a place, where you can bear your soul and say, '*I did not even see this. I missed this completely.*' And then you can start reconnecting again.

**~Elisabeth: You cannot do it on your own, but only in dialogue with others. And real dialogue requires equality, respect, humility, love and compassion.**

**^Angelique:** It's called, 'the teeth of our people's feelings'. Bit by bit, in whatever way is required at the time, we make sure that we're not making that person feel any guilt, shame or blame in order for them to get through that process.

**^Deborah:** They've already been hearing that shame and guilt. We're helping them to release that.

**~Elisabeth: How do the graduate parents help with the four core parental values?**

**~Jeanine:** Protecting children from danger, helping them to develop an independent future, helping them to have good relationships and respect for themselves and others.

**^Angelique:** In our group, there were a lot of safety issues and harm to the parents, and we had to get them to understand that it is a lot more serious when they're getting beaten up by their children than when their children are not putting their socks in a washing basket. It had to be voiced that they need to think about respect, safety and about connecting with their family members. They weren't getting it, until I explained about my situation with my son. And then they understood that, talking about my own child's safety was my input as a graduate parent, and that's when the penny dropped for a lot of the parents in our group.

**#Sukena:** One parent had a child who was looking at something very inappropriate: porn. She thought it was quite funny without thinking about the actual implication. We asked her, '*What if the school sees his phone and asks you about it? Would you still find that funny? It's not your son but you who is responsible.*' And she was quiet. It really impacted and resonated that you as a parent are responsible. And a lot of parents have a bit of a light bulb moment. We used it to highlight safety first.

***Carly:** It's about acknowledging it and putting it into practice.

**~Elisabeth: The values in NVR are used in a generic way to help prioritising positively rather than negatively that everybody can fit them to their own situation.**

**^Deborah:** I think the values help you to affirm why it's important what you're doing. Because by the time you get to NVR, you're usually in a place where you've almost forgotten about your values, where you're near to hitting your child. By having the values brought back to your attention, you realise, '*This is why I am there, why I am trying to find another solution to help my child*'.

**#Carly:** If the values are there, then comes respect; you learn to love them again and your whole family gets involved. It's working for me, because we've got the values and we're respecting each other, having pleasant times indoors. And we've not had that for a long time.

**~Dorota:** In my group we've got a few parents whose children are not violent and not expressive. Their problems are rather internalised; kids who wouldn't want to go to school or don't want to leave their room and plunge into depression. And still the values need to be resurrected.

**~Elisabeth: Haim Omer uses the phrase 'anchor function' that parents have for their children, keeping them in a safe haven. He uses it for parents. Does that also fit for what graduate parents do for new parents?**

**#Karina:** When it came to self-announcement, I was holding on to the guilt. It was so difficult. I felt like giving up. I felt like I couldn't cope any more with his behaviour and all the challenges, and I couldn't do it anymore. I was giving up, but I didn't want to. But that's how bad the situation was making me feel. So getting to the self-announcement and being able to say, '*I feel really guilty*'. And to let go of that, because doing NVR means 'connection before correction'. I realised that I wasn't present, that I was withdrawing myself from my child, from the situation, because I didn't like it. And if I wanted to make a correction to his behaviour I needed to connect first. And then it worked for me. I want to share that with other parents. So if I can tell this to other people and relate my situation to them, then I become their anchor.

**~Elisabeth: Michael White calls the process where people separate the problem from the person 'externalising'. 'Connection before correction' is how this is done in NVR.**

**^Sarah:** When I use 'connection before correction', I feel like I'm getting more of an understanding from my son. He opens up a lot more and I'm not judging him. I'm not blaming him, and it works a lot better for me. There is connection.

***Chinyere:** It's difficult to separate the child from the behaviour.

**#Sukaena:** I've noticed that parents like it when they hear about your situation, when you talk to them about NVR. It really encourages them. I didn't really understand the impact of 'striking, when the iron is cold'. As a parent, I always felt overwhelmed. You've got to be on top of everything, striking when the iron is hot over a pair of socks on the floor, whereas you could look at it, pick them up there and then and prioritise. I can now pass that on to other parents and tell them, '*How can we let that go and do something else?*'

**^Lesley:** With the connection I always go back to when the baby was first born. You don't expect the child to do anything. And neither do you correct them if they cry at the wrong time. You wouldn't dream of chastising a small baby. I mean, they just cry, and you have to accept it. You have to make that connection first. You're giving them unconditional love, no matter what they do as a baby. You just meet their needs. You just love them unconditionally, and you do whatever you have to do, and you don't expect anything back in return. And there are certain times in life when you have to go through that process. You do it when they are a baby. You do it when you're introducing someone else new into the family. And you do it again when they become teenagers or adults.

**~Pete:** We have quite a number of parents who have had quite difficult early experiences with their children and quite a lot of trauma.

**^Lesley:** They still have to make that connection later on. You always have an opportunity to make those connections, whether it be, when they are first born, six months old or four. You do have to make those connections.

**~Elisabeth: We have all come across hopelessness, despair, stuckness, blaming in new parents. When a new parent hits all your triggers and your trauma again, how do you, as graduate parent facilitators, manage to stay connected and not go back to where you have been and disconnect?**

**^Deborah:** Angelique once asked a parent who was doing her self-announcement key questions while sharing bits and pieces of her own testimony. You could see the light coming on: '*I can do this*'. And she wasn't able to do that without Angelique, who stayed grounded, while talking through her own trauma. The parent really connected because Angelique used her own story for the new parent's story.

**^Jacqui:** For me it would be going back to the baskets and saying, '*This is important. This is happening to somebody else now. And this is what needs to be looked after at present*'. And then put that first. That's how I follow through the stages. Yourself and things have improved or are improving. And the situation with somebody else at the present time is far worse or in a different place than where you are.

**#Karina:** Through completing the NVR process myself, I evolved as a person. And then I'm able, when someone else is talking about their trauma, not to think about my own trauma but to think about how I was in that place and now I am in a better place. So it can work, and I've got to pass that onto them. Because my mentality, my mindset and my beliefs, that it can work, remain in me, and because I've evolved as a person, I don't get drawn into their trauma, into how bad they feel and how bad I felt about myself, whenever I listen to somebody else talking. NVR has taught me new techniques.

**#Sukaena:** You are passing the baton. NVR helped me, and I want to pass that baton over. And when you pass that baton, there is that connection that you have with those parents. NVR is something that's digested and revisited. With the new parent's trauma, it's like a place where I draw support from the professionals and the supervision is paramount for the parents and for me. When I'm going through my own issues and hearing other people's, I have the support from the others who are more established or more experienced or just in a different place. You draw support from that, using the NVR tool of support. That is what they're there for. Showing others that, when we are doing support in NVR, everyone becomes your supporter. It becomes a continuing domino effect.

**^Angelique:** I mention to parents right at the beginning, '*I have been in this for five years*'. So I'm giving them a concept, an idea, that it doesn't stop now. The thing that I always say is that I eat, sleep and breathe NVR, meaning that I don't shut down. It is for every situation. My son's situation is always ongoing. I do not stop. No matter what age, no matter where he is at, I'm on it all the time. Generally, it is embedded in me.

**^Linda:** Originally I did the NVR programme for my daughter, my youngest. And at that point, my second youngest had already left home. But he is now back in my life as a 25-year-old with a drug problem, and I'm using NVR all over again with him. It does, as you say, continue.

**^Deborah:** It's a life style.

**~Elisabeth: You hear and see the parent facilitators give their testimony and experience them with your whole body. How is this different from reading a testimony or watching a video?**

***Chinyere:** I find it very helpful to listen to them, because they speak with authority. Obviously they've been involved in it and are often still going through it. And to hear them speak and go into detail, it brings it alive. You are there with that person. Because they're speaking from a place of experience. It's easier for you to imagine what they are saying, listen to what they're saying. They're more credible. Quotes that are read are also very helpful. But, I think, hearing it directly from the horse's mouth brings it to life that bit more.

***Carly:** When the parent facilitators are talking and telling us their stories they have a lot of compassion. But it also makes me feel relaxed about not being the only one in that position. And I don't feel judged at all, because they have lived it. They're living it out still now. So, I don't mind, talking about my experiences to them, and I don't feel bad about it.

**^Deborah:** It's common ground.

***Chinyere:** If they're going to open up and share that with you, then you feel more inclined to open up with them.

***Carly:** I'm a visual, face-to-face person. I remember receiving CBT once on the phone. I didn't enjoy it because I didn't know who I was talking to. And I couldn't put this voice to a face. So it's more heartfelt and more personal. I like the way that some stories are put with humour, some with great sadness. You feel everything, what they felt, a touch of it.

***Chinyere:** When you're talking, you're expressing, and when they're talking, they're also expressing. You can hear the emotion in their voices. Often they speak with passion. And every parent facilitator's story is different. And the way of dealing with it is different. So you know that this will be also true for you and for everybody else. So you just know that it's not a one size fits all. But you can draw strength from knowing that each person has found a way of dealing with it individually.

**~Elisabeth: When graduate parents are giving testimonies, the new parents are 'witnessing'.**

**~Jeanine:** My example of that insider witnessing comes from the graduation ceremony, where some people didn't feel ready to read out their own testimonies but had someone read them on their behalf. That process links with being an insider witness, when you see and hear their testimony.

**~Elisabeth: A zoologist called Adrian Thomas talked on the BBC about how his research on the flight behaviours of birds can be used for the development of drones in the military. He said, 'You do not copy the animal. You copy the design, the principal, of what it was intending to achieve'. How do you link that to your own situations?**

***Chinyere:** You don't know how you're going to get on with what they say it is supposed to do. You try it out and then see the results for yourself.

**^Deborah:** You get your own experience from trying out the tools and the information that you receive. And that's what develops your story. Because each story changes. Each person who comes to NVR doesn't have the same story. You have similar situations, but your story will still be different. But the tools that enable you to get to or to overcome each challenge are the same. But how you adapt them will be different. I tell parents, '*NVR is like getting a driving license. Once you get your license, you use it as and when. Sometimes I walk, sometimes I take the bus. I don't always use my car, but if I need to get somewhere quicker, I will use my car. And I will use whatever NVR tools are within my reach.*'

**~Elisabeth: So, you are also saying, 'Even in my own set of behaviours, I don't copy the one tool that I learnt, in exactly the same way. We re-design each time'.**

**^Deborah:** That's exactly why NVR has evolved to where it is. The work books have changed, have been adapted and have been reconstructed from each experience.

**~Elisabeth: So there is a design behind it rather than just content.**

**Deborah:** A plane is not going like a bird, but is designed to be able to fly.

**~Elisabeth: Deborah, you also used the metaphor of the cake, seeing 'Bake Off' on television and wanting to copy it?**

 

**^Deborah:** I was using the same ingredients, but if you added them differently, at a different time with a different temperature, it would come out differently.

**~Elisabeth: Are there situations where parent participation may be counter-productive?**

**#Karina:** My children don't go to the school where I am facilitating but there are some parents who do facilitate at their children's school, and where there may be a conflict between their children and the school. That is quite difficult. Or seeing another mum in the playground who you are in parent support with and who you don't want to know your story and your business. That can be a little bit of a barrier. Or if you are from the same very connected community and know each other's family and friends, that can be a barrier. Maybe some parents don't want to share their information with you because there is a connection between you.

**~Elisabeth: You're all so enthusiastic. You want to help, but how much can you do? Who can you do it with? In which situation could you put yourself or others in danger?**

**^Lesley:** I think there are quite a lot of parent facilitators who need more help with boundaries, perhaps even before becoming parent facilitators. They need to be involved in some discussion around where and when you do parent facilitating. I know somebody who has chosen not to volunteer in this area. She travels to another borough from hers because she doesn't want to be in the same area as her child, sharing stories about her child, about what is private or personal. She said, '*It's my daughter's story, and I'm telling everybody my daughter's story, as well as my mine. I don't want to do that in this area, so I'll go somewhere else and do it there*'.

**~Jeanine:** And as a school, maybe, we should use parent facilitators whose children have already left the school or who are coming back a year after. Or work with parents of much older children who are put in with parents of Year 7 students (aged 11–12 years), so that there's a big enough gap between the children.

**^Lesley:** There needs to be a bit more thought about that, more discussion. Everybody is so enthusiastic.

**~Pete:** We have to be sensitive. If there's a parent facilitator who has the same child in the same school as a new parent on the course, how do we discuss that? Does that feel OK or not? Supervision is the key.

**~Elisabeth: What have you learnt about yourselves in the process?**

***Alison:** When I first started NVR I couldn't see the purpose of it at all. Dorota asked me to turn up, and I did. And I just sat there and thought, '*My son doesn't hit me or anything like that ... I'm not going to fit in here. I don't know if it's going to work. I'll give it another week*'. And at the end, I said, '*I still don't think it really relates, but at least I've got the tools to put in my pocket*'. But going back again this year there's someone in the group who is in the same position as me then, and I could just read her straight away.

**#Karina:** Alison used to be bored. Now she's a graduate parent, and a new parent, who doesn't want to be there, really relates to her. Alison makes that parent want to come back.

**^Angelique:** It's taught me that I've got a lot of other strengths that I never knew I had.

**^Linda**: My confidence, self-confidence, has really improved. Just knowing that you can do things. I think when you have difficulties in the family with the children, it knocks your self-confidence. You feel a failure. You can't get anything right. So to go through all these processes, and then go on and help other parents is boosting your confidence. It really boosted my self-esteem and helped me get a job at the end of it.

**^Deborah:** I think what I learned from NVR is that it's an ongoing lifestyle. I sometimes draw strength from talking to the other graduate parents. It's a lifetime of networking. We're connected through NVR. I've learnt that NVR is a connecting tool, and not just with my child.

**^Sarah:** What I got from it is keeping NVR fresh in my head. Because when you've just done that once in the group it's easy to go back to your old ways. But by being a parent facilitator, it stays with you.

***Carly:** It's like a refresher.

**^Sarah:** And you're adding to the group.

**^Deborah:** And you're learning more.

**~Elisabeth: How can the participatory approach be extended in NVR groups and beyond? Can you imagine it with individual NVR?**

 

**~Jane:** I think so. I remember doing home visits before the specialist group with a graduate parent. I wouldn't have been able to get through the door without the graduate parent there. I think if there's someone who's especially fragile and not able to access the group at that time, it would be a very useful approach to have a professional and a graduate parent working on a one-family-basis, maybe with a view that they might eventually join a group. It had made a massive difference in how the families engaged.

**~Elisabeth: What would you recommend to people who want to implement participatory practice in NVR?**

**^Deborah:** Give it a go. Try it, there is no harm in trying!

**^Linda:** You never know until you try it.

***Alison:** Don't give up! Keep going!

***Ashley:** You've got to complete it. If you don't complete it, it's not going to mean anything.

**^Lesley:** Participate in two groups with graduate parents first because you all need to learn to work with each other. Start with parents who are quite sure of their role, even with different people. Work with somebody at least twice! Professionals also need to know that they need to support their parent facilitators. It's two-way.

**~Dorota:** We're using NVR on ourselves because we need to be able to connect. How can we NVR each other and effectively support each other?

**~Elisabeth: Is there anything we have missed out?**

**^Deborah:** I'm grateful for the acknowledgment of our role. If it wasn't acknowledged or recognised we'd not be where we are. We were all in a place of 'rock bottom' with different stories. It helped me to regain my confidence, my boldness, and say to myself: *'I'm taking this on. I am going to resist. I am going to persist'*. A whole new world opened up for me. From just doing a tick box exercise, it just evolved. And now I have permanent connections that are never going to crumble for me.

**~Jeanine:** How do we get male graduate parents as a resource to reach out to other parents?

**^Lesley:** Most of the time the men are working.

^**Angelique:** In a lot of the groups, the men who do come often say straight away, *'I can come for a few sessions, but not to all. I have got to go to work.'* That's quite common. Do something separate from what we've got already.

*__Carly:__ The process is much faster when you're together.

^**Deborah:** Spouses should get a taster session – a couple of hours or a condensed session for one day. When they say they can't make it, they're working, you can point out that it's just one session, where you are pulling and drawing in all the key NVR things.

~**Jeanine:** And address with them, *'How is what you are going to learn today helping you to support the person who comes weekly?'*

^**Lesley:** It's really a case of encouraging them to come. How are we going to get them to a place without making them feel awkward? We have to meet them where they are.

^**Deborah:** There's the male pride issue. My husband is over 50; if there's a young facilitator, he'd be thinking, *'She's never going to tell me what to do. I've had eight children. How many has she had?'* That would be in the back of his mind.

~**Jeanine:** When referrals come through, think about who's in the network and who are the key people, whether it is a dad, an uncle, a grandparent, a neighbour. Who needs to be involved?

^**Lesley:** It's about how we can get to them. How, where and when we do it.

~**Elisabeth: What was the most important thing about graduate parents' participation that we discussed today?**

^**Lesley:** That brings us back to the beginning. We are the bridge between the parents and the professionals.

^**Deborah:** We keep it real.

^**Angelique:** We all support each other, because we still have things going on in our lives and our journey. We all stay connected, and that connection is getting across to the groups that we end up facilitating. They can feel that.

~**Jane:** We were thinking about a motto like glue before. I now think of the word 'cement', they actually 'cement' NVR.

^**Deborah:** It was the acknowledgement of what we are and add to the group.

**~Elisabeth: Are you now more aware of the added value that you bring to NVR?**

*__Ashley:__ I'm glad I came. Because it's just good to be around people who've been through the same thing. I'm so grateful to have the opportunity to do this NVR course.

*__Chinyere:__ I'm glad I came as well. Because I've learnt some things that I didn't understand before. What people have said has helped me to understand what I have learnt so far and consolidate it more.

*__Carly:__ I feel slightly more educated in NVR, and it has refreshed everything again.

^**Deborah:** I'm glad I came. Today has made me excited again that NVR isn't phasing out. If anything it's alive and kicking and well and going into new dimensions with new people, which is brilliant.

^**Sarah:** And it's forever growing.

**~Elisabeth: Thank you all very much for your contributions!**

# Chapter 18: Expanding reconciliation gestures and active resistance with connecting and resisting comments

**By Pete Brown**

## Introduction

Reconciliation gestures and active resistance are important ideas in non-violent resistance (NVR), and they can be seen as two sides of the same coin. The essence of these ideas can be captured by the saying 'connection before correction' – on the one hand, reconciliation gestures emphasise connection, while active resistance emphasises correction. 'Resisting comments' replace the word 'correction' in NVR as this creates a better fit with the ethos of *resistance* in the NVR programme.

In this chapter I will suggest that a selection of pre-planned comments, called connecting comments and resisting comments, can be very helpful as stepping stones to re-building the relationship between parent and child. We have been experimenting with these ideas on the NVR parent courses that I organise two to three times a year. Parents' comments about aspects of their impact are shown in the appendix.

These ideas come from social learning and systemic theory, as well as narrative ideas within the systemic field. I suggest that connecting and resisting comments offer an initial structured starting point that parents and carers can then adapt as relationships improve. It is therefore suggested that pre-planned comments are helpful near the start of the NVR programme when parents are in a high state of stress and the prospect of escalation is ever present.

Both connecting and resisting comments focus on the significance of language and words. I am mindful that spaces between words are also important. Other reconciliation gestures of shared time together (Omer, 2004, p70), reflective listening and vigilant care (Omer, 2017, p42) are present in our NVR programme, but beyond the scope of this chapter.

Woven through the fabric of this chapter is the notion of 'a difference that makes a difference', from Bateson (1972) and expanded upon by Andersen (1987), in what I call the 'Goldilocks zone of change' (which I will explain further on). This is brought together with ideas of timing, tone and talk (adapted from Taylor, 2010).

## The importance of carefully choosing our words

> *Sticks and stones may break my bones but words will never hurt me.*

Contrary to the above saying, words *can* hurt. Families often get locked into negative and vicious verbal battles and we frequently come across parents who feel deeply wounded by their children's hurtful comments. A common one, at the milder end of the spectrum, is '*I hate you – you are a terrible mother/father*'.

Some children and young people become very adept at making provocative, negative comments. Introducing a selection of pre-prepared connecting and resisting comments is part of a two-part recipe for improving verbal communication and developing the potential of dialogues to move beyond problem-saturated discourses that have led to an impasse in the parent-child relationship (White & Epston, 1990).

Creating a range of these comments arose from questions raised on NVR parent courses about what to do after learning how to de-escalate. 'Strike while the iron is cold' is a powerful motto of NVR, but many parents often then ask, '*what do we say when the iron is cold?*'

Omer (2004, p69) mentions verbal reconciliation gestures but they are not discussed in detail. In a later work, he suggests that it is the *regular contact* of parent and child that helps to increase parental presence (Omer, 2017). However, greater contact can also lead to an increased risk of escalation; hence these tools can be very helpful in beginning to support calmer encounters.

 

## Timing, tone and talk

For both connecting and resisting comments we introduce the idea of 'timing, tone and talk', adapted from the educationalist Taylor (2010). Each of these helps parents to structure an interaction, letting them consider *when to talk* (timing), *how to say it* (tone) and *what to say* (talk). Delayed reactions as well as planned actions are central ideas in NVR. The first two 't's remind parents of the importance of neutral times and neutral tones. The third 't', talk, refers to the pre-planned comments that I will shortly describe.

## Comments vs conversations

In considering connecting and resisting comments, it is important to remember that these are indeed comments rather than conversations. They are short, succinct comments that can lead to improved conversations, but they are necessarily brief at the start of this process where the risk of escalation is high. As the comments become more familiar, they can lead to richer, warmer, longer conversations over time.

## The need for pre-planned comments

Pre-planned comments can be very helpful early in the NVR process. As most spontaneous comments invariably lead to escalation, parents are offered a selection of pre-rehearsed comments, stripped back of the blaming aspects of language, and with 'ingredients' that may help conversations to run more smoothly.

It is useful to draw a distinction between impulsive and planned comments. Impulsive comments tend to be corrective, critical statements, usually delivered in the heat of the moment and often tarnished with insults or reprimands. Pre-planned and rehearsed comments gradually introduce differences that help connections to occur. As parental presence returns, parents are gradually more able to judge when to use immediate or delayed comments, and better able to predict how these will be received by the child.

Readers familiar with NVR ideas will see the similarity here with 'the announcement', which is a pre-rehearsed, pre-prepared and written script delivered to children at a neutral time to address one or two very serious issues (known as 'small basket' behaviours). The connecting and resisting comments can be seen as experiments with less escalatory conversations before the introduction of the more formal announcement. Some parents have called these 'mini-announcements'. Parents on our courses have also reported that the connecting and resisting comments can assist with finding appropriate words when preparing The Announcement.

The idea of pre-planned comments can sit uncomfortably with practitioners who prefer a less prescriptive stance. Many parents have asked for a selection of comments because they report feeling stuck in their current patterns of interaction. It can be difficult to think clearly in highly stressed and emotionally charged situations. I suggest that pre-planned comments that offer an overall collaborative stance help to support parents under stress to improve communication.

I am influenced by the notion of 'authoritative doubt', which I think can lead to a position of both 'expert' and 'collaborator' (Mason, 2010). We may offer ideas from a position of authority, more or less, but the way we impart these ideas should be collaborative and should include space for the parent's voice and ideas. Many of my ideas have been influenced by parental feedback and I see these ideas as a still-emerging approach.

## Connecting comments

> *'When I make a mistake, no one forgets; when I do well, no one sees.'*
> (Severe, 2000)

Hedges (2010) notes that up to 90% of comments given by parents to children can be negative. Most parents who come to the course are also experts in self-criticism. Parents are invariably caught up in a pattern of blaming the child and themselves. One parent at the start of the NVR parent course called it the 'failed parents club'.

Flaskas (2011, p91) suggests that there is broad agreement within the systemic field of the value of a strengths based ethos. This runs from the earlier days of 'positive connotation' to the current post-modern approaches that emphasise use of language and the co-construction of meaning through dialogue.

As we introduce NVR ideas to parents and carers, we search for and try to notice the strengths available to them. From a narrative perspective, we search for 'unique outcomes' of parental changes. These changes usually take place in a slow, uneven way as parents experiment with creating small differences. Brookfield (2015) talks of a learning process as '*two steps forward and one step back*'. This idea has proven helpful for parents who may feel reassured to hear that backwards steps can be followed by forward steps, then backwards and forwards again, within an overall process of slow, incremental forward progress. It helps to sustain a feeling of realistic hope, although there can be frustration that changes happen over-time rather than over-night.

In looking at the process of change, I am influenced by Bateson's (1972) passage, often quoted within systems theory: '*a difference that makes a difference*'. Andersen's (1987, p2) ideas about introducing difference build on this, as he proposes three kinds of linguistic difference that are important to consider:

> '*The first is a difference that is too small to be noticed by the recipient. The second is an appreciable difference, meaning that it is big enough to be noticed. The third is a difference that is too great and may have a disorganising effect on the system.*'

Flaskas (2011) notes that Tom Andersen's ideas move well beyond the concept of dialogue-in-language to also include language-of-the-body and emotionally attuned practices. I acknowledge these important ideas even though they are beyond the scope of this chapter.

I call these ideas – 'too much difference', 'too little difference' and 'just the right amount of difference' – the 'Goldilocks zone of change' after the classic *Goldilocks and the three bears* fairy-tale (Brown, 2019).

We can link these ideas to timing, tone and talk to ensure the connecting and resisting comments fall within the Goldilocks' zone of 'the right amount of difference'.

## Introducing the 'magnifying glass'

As we introduce connecting comments, we encourage parents to actively look for the exceptions to their own children's problematic attitudes and behaviours. As this can be challenging at the start of the NVR process we use the metaphor of a magnifying glass. On the parenting course we bring in an actual magnifying glass to illustrate the point. This idea fits well with the concept of the baskets, and we link it to the idea of the rainbow basket – the basket where parents place things that they like about their child, but which have become lost under the weight of difficult issues. Our aim is to re-kindle lost connections and bring these into sight, or into sharper focus. As I have said elsewhere, '*Quite often, behind a very serious argument, is often a lot of missed opportunities for love, caring, concern about each other, which is still there, but very much under the surface.*' (Brown, 2013)

# Six ideas about the use of pre-planned connecting comments

I will now explain some connecting comments that we offer parents and include some advice for using them. Some of these originate in a variety of parenting texts, based on social learning theory (e.g. Webster-Stratton, 2006; Taylor, 2010; Janis-Norton, 2016) but all, in my view, need adaptations for use within an NVR framework.

In most parenting literature, attention is given to the importance of positive feedback, and the phrase '*catch the child being good*' is often used. This is a far better approach than punishment based approaches, which in my clinical experience, are still widely used by many parents and teachers.

However, the terms 'praise' and 'positive feedback' are often associated with a behaviourist approach. I have therefore opted to use the term 'appreciation', as I think this creates a clearer link to the notion of relationships and the idea of 'doing with' rather than 'doing to'. Also, most parenting literature (usually aimed at parents of children in young or middle childhood) emphasises the importance of giving enthusiastic praise. For the ideas given below there is a general adaptation of using more neutral tones and less overt enthusiasm when imparting comments of appreciation. Not only is this is more appropriate for older children and teenagers, but it also fits with the Goldilocks idea of introducing small appreciable differences that are less likely to be rejected when making inroads into problem-saturated discourses.

As I see these pre-planned comments as stepping stones to eventually richer conversations and dialogue, I also wish to emphasise that these can be developed by parents as they gain more confidence.

1. **Low key greetings:** The first type of connecting comment that we suggest are simply 'low key greeting comments'. We ask parents to avoid adding any other comments at all (as these invariably become criticisms at this early stage of change). For example, they might say, *'Hi, good to see you'*, or, *'Morning, breakfast is ready'* but then 'bite their lip' if they feel like adding any critical comment. After these types of comments we suggest that parents experiment with adding comments that show appreciation around areas of co-operation as I will outline below. The main idea here is to model polite and calm words and resist the tendency to match the child's hostility with parental hostility.
2. **Descriptive appreciation:** This simply means using words to describe our comments, so that they become specific rather than general. 'Descriptive appreciation' is useful for comments with all children, but especially children with some neuro-developmental conditions. For example, a general

Appreciative comment might be, '*Thanks for doing what I asked you*', while a descriptive appreciation could extend to, '*I appreciate your effort to go into school this morning*'.

3. **Subtle appreciation:** In my clinical experience, low-key subtle appreciation is generally more appropriate, and less likely to be rejected, by older children and adolescents, as well as children with more sensitive or intense temperaments including those diagnoses such as autistic spectrum condition and/or ADHD. For example, '*Thanks for coming in at the time I asked you to*' delivered in a low key way. (This is similar to adopting a neutral tone of voice; the difference is, in itself, subtle, perhaps using a quieter voice and inconspicuously dropping the appreciation into the sentence).

4. **Delayed appreciation:** Running counter to much of the parenting literature, we ask parents to be mindful of the timing of comments. We note that the use of 'delayed appreciation' can be very effective in helping children and young people to accept appreciative and strength-based comments. For example, '*I meant to say earlier, thanks for coming in at the time I asked you to*'.

5. **Combining appreciation and criticism:** This important tip is to remind parents and carers of what NOT to do after giving an appreciative comment. A well-known common pitfall is to add criticism after appreciation. This tendency has the effect of leaving the recipient with a sour taste of correction that cancels out the earlier appreciation. For example, '*Thanks for coming in at the time I asked you to. If you did this every time, wouldn't life be easier?*' A variation of this, also to be avoided, is to combine appreciation with a reminder. For example, '*Thanks for coming in at the time I asked you to. I hope you will do this again tomorrow*'. While often well meaning, in practice I have seen time and again young people interpret the reminder as a criticism, cancelling out the earlier comment of appreciation.

6. **3-1 appreciation strategy:** The last piece of advice that I would like to address in this section on appreciation comments, is asking parents to consider the ratio of 'connection' to 'correction' comments, or, to put it another way, 'the 3-1 appreciation vs criticism strategy' (adapted from Taylor, 2010). Interestingly, we find that this ratio often stays in parents' minds and helps them to stay silent when they feel compelled to offer critical comments. It also helps to recognise that current conversations are usually saturated with arguments and reprimands. The premise here is simply that connecting ways of talking are always more powerful when it comes to improving the parent-child relationship and increasing parental presence. The 3-1 recipe provides a very concrete reminder of the importance of connecting conversations. (Over time, an aim is to reach Taylor's suggestion of a 6-1 strategy, but clinical experience shows this is usually too ambitious in the early days of working on small yet significant changes. Additionally, the level of change can move beyond the Goldilocks zone and create 'too much difference' if introduced too quickly).

The above comments and advice are like a recipe. For a new recipe, we usually stick to the instructions. However, as we become more familiar, we may vary the recipe and make useful adaptations, and even improvements. I have noticed that as family relationships improve, parents do incorporate the pre-planned appreciation comments into their own conversational dialogues that become richer and more ambitious over time. This happens as the connection with their child increases and their parental presence returns.

Parents are warned that children and young people will sometimes impart scathing responses to these initial comments and will not usually return any comments of appreciation, although this does tend to change, little by little over time. When children reject or belittle appreciative comments, it can be helpful to imagine a shield of parental armour to protect oneself. I will say more about this in the next section. And when things do change, often in very small ways, efforts by the child should not go unnoticed. Parents are usually so relieved when there are calm moments, that it is often easier not to comment on any improvements. However it is precisely at these calmer, neutral times that connecting comments should be given. In other words, comments of appreciation can be given at 'strike while the iron is cold' moments – not only resisting comments, which we will look at shortly.

Perseverance is fundamental as parents begin to change the currency of conversations in these subtle but important ways. I am convinced, through my clinical experience, that calling attention to strengths, with regular comments of appreciation and encouragement, paying attention to timing, tone and talk, will slowly and steadily improve parent-child relationships. I have noticed that parents often begin to notice changes in themselves as they de-escalate and use more polite and calm connecting and resisting comments. As they feel better about their own actions and reactions, a reflexive process of mutual change between parent and child can develop over time.

## Summary

Just as practitioners try to build slowly on what parents do well, and notice attempts to make small changes, we ask parents to experiment in a similar fashion, by using a metaphorical magnifying glass to help notice seeds of strengths in their children and, just as importantly, comment on them using pre-planned appreciative comments. The pre-planned comments may then eventually give way to richer dialogues, over time.

 

# Resisting comments and statements

*'What you resist, persists'* (Carl Jung)

Giving verbal corrections is difficult. Verbal corrections can easily turn into angry arguments. Sometimes parents can become caught in a pattern of withdrawal as a way of avoiding arguments. Omer (2017) talks of strengthening parental presence in the child's mind when there is routine contact with the child. He suggests it is a parental duty to maintain contact and to make regular enquiries about the child (such as their whereabouts, behaviour, computer habits etc).

Resisting comments also pay attention to timing, tone and talk, and are not imparted as criticisms, reprimands or insults given when the parent is angry or frustrated. As with connecting comments, they are carefully thought through and pre-planned statements, given whenever possible at neutral times using the 'cold iron' approach. The ideas of these statements come mainly from systemic and narrative therapy that introduce the possibilities of change in a respectful way and within the 'not too different' and 'not too similar' Goldilocks zone of change.

There is surprisingly little in the parenting literature about how to give corrective yet respectful statements. When we talk with parents we pose the question, '*how do you address issues, without squashing your child's spirit?*' Once parents agree that their children are very frequently criticised, often in school as well as home, they will usually agree that it would be helpful to find a better and less blaming way to talk to them.

## Six ideas about the use of pre-planned resisting comments

For all of the following statements, I suggest they be short and succinct. They are not one-off conversations, but short statements that will frequently be revisited to continue to show active resistance and increase parental presence. Resisting comments, under the umbrella of active resistance, help the parent to address rather than avoid issues in non-escalatory ways. Some of these ideas are often employed by therapists to facilitate difficult conversations and can quite easily be adapted for use by parents.

1. **Adding an introductory sentence:** In systemic literature, Burnham (2005) states that prefacing comments 'warm the context' and help subsequent comments to follow more smoothly. For example, '*I don't think this will be easy for either of us, but I'd like to talk briefly about something that has been worrying me*'.

2. **Making an appointment:** A survey conducted some years ago showed an aspect that young people dislike more than anything else – spontaneous problem solving parental lectures (Phelan, 1998). In my experience, making an appointment often works surprisingly well. For example, *'I'd like to talk about this later, after dinner, when we have both had a chance to calm down'*. The following example combines an introductory sentence with the suggestion of an appointment: *'I want to talk about something that is worrying me. Do you want to talk now or later at, say, 7pm?'*
3. **Combining an appreciative element to the statement:** Appreciation and criticism should never be combined, as discussed earlier, but it is possible to do the reverse; that is, add appreciation after a resisting comment. For example, *'I'm concerned that you didn't go into school today. I've noticed you have made a real effort to get into school more often'*
4. **Using 'I' and point of view statements rather than 'you' statements:** The origin of 'I' statements is difficult to ascertain, but they appear to have come from Carl Rogers and the humanistic approach. 'You' statements are very common, especially from parents to children. Having observed these over many years, I can see they easily evoke defences in the recipient. However, a slight shift of words makes a lot of difference in gaining co-operation. For example, *'I'd like you to come home by 10pm, please'* instead of, *'You need to come home by 10pm'*. Point of view statements change a 'hard fact' into a 'point of view', and these are usually better received by older children and young people in situations of conflict. One simply adds: *'From my point of view…' 'The way I see it is…' 'You may disagree, but from my perspective…' 'You may not like this, but I feel that...'* To use the above example this would then look like, *'You may not agree, but from my point of view I'd like to you to come home by 10pm'*.

   Many parents are concerned that these sorts of statements can leave the child or young person with the impression that the request is optional. This is not the intention. The idea is to use assertive yet polite language that increases parental presence by creating a sentence with the aim of encouraging co-operation when there is usually no co-operation. These comments help to side-step the risk of escalation, which is often only seconds away. And when escalation occurs, non-cooperation is guaranteed.
5. **Maintaining a problem focus, not a person focus:** This powerful and enduring idea from narrative therapy should not be underestimated. This helps parents to avoid an often retaliatory stance of 'name calling'. I regard name-calling as very damaging to self-esteem. I gave an example of a typical comment from a child to parent earlier in this chapter. A typical comment from a parent to child, also from the milder end, is *'Why are you so stupid? Anyone who would do that is an idiot.'* Narrative therapy makes clear that 'the problem is the problem' (White & Epston,1990), not the person. With this in mind, parents are always encouraged to criticise the behaviour, not the child. When the problem is viewed as external to the child, it becomes easier

 

to change. The example below shows another linguistic shift from 'I' to 'We' statements. This focuses the issue as a family problem, rather than something intrinsic to the child. For example, '*This is a problem that we need to think about more*' or '*We need to loosen the grip of this problem*'.

6. **Prefacing comments as a parental duty:** There is something about 'parental duty' statements that even children with the most oppositional behaviour will accept if given at neutral times, in neutral tones, and with neutral talk. Omer (2017) gives helpful examples of parental duty comments, including ideas that help promote vigilant care in the face of children masking and hiding worrying issues. For example, '*I know this isn't pleasant for you, but it's my parental duty to not let you stay on the computer all night. It's my duty to make sure it's turned off at a reasonable time, so that you get enough sleep.*'

A mix-and-match approach to these comments can be taken. The following example blends an 'I' statement and a parental duty statement: '*You may disagree but I would like you to come home by 10pm. It's my parental duty to request that you come home by this time please*'.

Connecting and resisting comments have much in common with Weinblatt's guides to 'recovering conversations'. I consider his guiding sentences as similar to connecting and resisting comments, and possibly a merger of them. A difference is that he offers these guides for the NVR 'sit-in' conversations (Weinblatt, 2015).

With all of these statements, the child or young person can easily react explosively or pleadingly or alternate between various positions. I find that *without parental reaction*, this can calm down quickly much of the time. Hence the importance of the metaphorical 'shield' to protect the parent from retaliation, mutual escalation or a pattern of withdrawing.

## Introducing the 'shield'

The above tips for making statements help resisting comments to go that bit more smoothly, but as many parents will testify, they do not guarantee the child will respond in a calm way. This is where the idea of 'the shield' is introduced. This is simply a metaphor for an imaginary protective screen, or parental armour, to help parents manage a child's hostile reactions to this feedback. Resisting comments (and indeed connecting comments) will often be met with initial hostility or contempt.

The Shield helps parents to feel less wounded by hurtful comments and also supports a non-retaliatory stance. On the NVR course, I bring in a fireguard to illustrate the point; this often fills the room with knowing, tense laughter as parents see the analogy of the child's heated, fiery comments met by the fireguard or shield. (This idea arose from doing trauma work, where a metaphorical shield may be used to support a journey through traumatic material). It is important to note that the shield is 'one-way armour'. Parents raise the imaginary shield to protect themselves from insults, but then lower it to maintain a connection with the child. This is a difficult stance that becomes easier to manage over time.

## Conclusion

Once parents become familiar with these ideas, practice is needed. I explain that both connecting and resisting comments are always easier to talk about than to put into practice (Nichols, 2013, personal communication). I find the following systemic equation from Mason (2010) very helpful in supporting parents to experiment with creating these changes in the Goldilocks zone of 'a difference that makes a difference'.

Change = a commitment to experimenting with difference + action + repetition + time

Parents have commented on the amount of mental and emotional effort needed in terms of self-discipline, self-control and self-awareness to maintain NVR practice over time. Sometimes there are leaps of progress, although it is more common to find a 'two steps forward, one step back' progression of change as discussed earlier. Here is my adaptation of the above equation.

Change = a commitment to experimenting with difference + action + repetition + mental and emotional effort + time

---

*Feeling more comfortable with feeling uncomfortable as change takes place*

The second part of the equation – 'feeling more comfortable with feeling uncomfortable' – is based on parental feedback gained from NVR parent courses. As the course progresses and NVR ideas become more familiar, parents and carers usually report a growing confidence of living with the tension of creating these small, yet significant differences.

As time goes on and parental presence is regained, a mixed approach to connecting and resisting comments often takes place. Richer conversations and encounters happen more often. As NVR becomes part of a parent's repertoire, both rehearsal and spontaneity become more merged with comments delivered with an increasing air of non-escalatory confidence. Ultimately, these ideas all have the purpose of seeing the child more clearly, connecting very often, resisting very often, regaining parental presence and rebuilding the parent-child relationship.

# Appendix

Here is some feedback from parents and carers about the use of pre-planned connecting and resisting comments (taken following a 12-week NVR parent course, Autumn 2017 – Spring 2018).

- *I find by striking while the iron is cold my son will listen to me rather than just dismissing me. I also rehearse my words carefully, using a polite but constructive manner.*
- *When my son is calm, I get my point across, and try the pre-planned comments. When he's angry I've learnt not to respond.*
- *Timing is important, especially when needing to discuss any inappropriate behaviour. I use little, calm, planned statements and even these are very difficult for her to hear.*
- *Strike while the iron is cold is essential and I am now able to do this on most occasions and take time to plan how I will approach certain situations. I use more delayed comments and say thank you for certain things i.e. when my daughter has tidied up.*
- *The ideas are helpful to put things in perspective with tone, timing and talk. I have been silent when abusive comments start. They have not stopped, but they have been less.*
- *I like the recommended frequency of appreciation to criticism. I use pre-planned conversations to discuss stealing.*
- *Instead of telling my child that she has done a silly thing and that was stupid, I've changed my delivery of the conversation and guide her to a more positive way of dealing with situations.*
- *The shield helps me to feel less hurt by some of the appalling comments thrown at me. If I can refrain from answering back, the storm passes more quickly.*
- *I use the shield to protect myself from my son's hostile insults. I now need to focus on the magnifying glass.*
- *The subtle appreciation has been helpful with my younger son in getting him to reflect on his strengths and, with computers, work responsibly and stick to time limits.*
- *I have used most of the connecting conversation ideas, but found that using 'I' statements are most beneficial to my children as they seem to feel that I nag less than before.*

# References

Andersen T (1987) The Reflecting Team: Dialogue and Meta-Dialogue in Clinical Work. *Family Process* **26** 415–428.

Bateson G (1972) *Steps to an Ecology of Mind*. University of Chicago press.

Burnham J (2005) *Relational Reflexivity: A tool for socially constructing therapeutic relationships*. In: C Flaskas, B Mason & A Perlesz (eds) The Space Between: Experience, context, and process in the therapeutic relationship. Karnac Books.

Brookfield S (2015) *The Skilful Teacher*. Jossey-Bass.

Brown P (2013) Using Reflecting Role Plays in Reflecting Teams. *Context Magazine*, April 2013. AFT Publishing.

Brown P (2019) Working therapeutically in the Goldilocks Zone. *Context Magazine*, due for publication February 2019. AFT Publishing.

Day EM & Heismann E (2010) *Non-Violent Resistance Programme: For all those working with parents and carers of children and adolescents with violent behaviours*. Pavilion Publishing.

Flaskas C (2011) Frameworks for Practice in the Systemic Field. Part 2 – Contemporary Frameworks in Family Therapy. *Australian and New Zealand Journal of Family Therapy* **32** (2) pp87–108.

Hedges F (2010) *Reflexivity in Therapeutic Practice*. Palgrave Macmillian.

Janis-Norton N (2015) *Calmer, Easier, Happier Boys*. YellowKite books.

Mason B (2010) 'Some ideas about the nature of therapy: a professional history re-visited'. In: TB Huat & C Lim (eds) *Journeys in Systemic Psychotherapy: Theory, practice and research*. Singapore. Armour Publishing.

Nichols R (2013) Personal communication while running an NVR course at Memorial Hospital, London, Oxleas NHS Trust.

Omer H (2004) *Nonviolence Resistance: A new approach to violent and self-destructive children.* Cambridge: Cambridge University Press.

Omer H (2017) *Parental Vigilant Care: A guide for clinicians and caretakers*. Routledge.

Phelan T (1998) *Surviving your Adolescents*. Parent magic, inc.

Severe S (2000) *How to Behave so Your Children will too*. Viking.

Taylor C (2010) *Divas and Door Slammers*. Vermilion.

Weinblatt U (2015) *Two-day NVR workshop.* Oxleas NHS Trust. Woolwich Centre, London, UK.

Webster-Stratton C (2006) *The Incredible Years*. Incredible Years.

White M & Epston D (1990) *Narrative Means to Therapeutic Ends*. Norton.

 

# Part 5: Working in and with schools

# Chapter 19: Non-violent resistance in and with schools

**By Dorota Rospierska & Kyla Evans**

## Introduction

This chapter takes a practical stance with the aim of illustrating what has been most useful in developing NVR parenting groups in schools and NVR practices among school staff. It describes how a team of parent and professional NVR facilitators have introduced and cultivated a discourse of NVR in large South East London secondary schools. It also discusses ideas about how to introduce new practices in parent-child relationships via NVR multifamily programs, and makes suggestions for exposing school staff to NVR language, concepts and behaviours. Links between the NVR approach and systemic theory and practice are made. It includes contributions from school staff and both parent and professional facilitators. We hope that it allows the reader to taste the richness of the NVR work we undertake.

## Setting the scene

> *'Reconciliation gestures in a classroom or around can be as simple as greeting every student at the door or positively commenting on their uniform, bag, hair style, work. This is practically simple to do and requires little planning time of planning which is perfect for teachers who are rushed off their feet.'*
> Head of Year at a secondary school

For those who are not familiar with the UK education system, secondary schools typically consist of around 1,300 pupils and over 200 staff. UK mental health services are increasingly integrating into community sites, such that schools are now expected to provide emotional and behavioural support as active parts of their communities, including offering help to parents and carers.

A report by the Department for Education (2016, p24) states that, *'evidence shows that if parents/carers can be supported to better manage their children's behaviour, alongside work being carried out with the child at school, there is a much greater likelihood of success in reducing the child's problems, and in supporting their academic and emotional development'*. In Greenwich, a London borough, Child and Adolescent Mental Health (CAMHS) link workers from Oxleas NHS Foundation Trust have been based in schools to fulfil these expectations.

This chapter describes the process whereby a CAMHS link worker used the NVR multi-families programme, based on the Oxleas NVR group programme (Day & Heismann, 2010), in order to achieve these aims. The family therapist and experienced NVR facilitator considered the approach to fit with the needs of parents and teachers who often raised concerns about pupils' volatile or violent behaviours towards parents, staff and peers. Self-destructive acts of hurting oneself and other risky behaviours including school refusal were frequent reasons for referral to the CAMHS link worker as a mental health professional within school.

School staff were invited to become trainee facilitators and organisers, giving them an opportunity for professional growth and skill development transferable to their relationship with pupils and colleagues. Through this process, an NVR schools community was established, which will be referred to in the rest of this chapter as 'we'.

## Theory and literature – links to systemic thinking

There is some well-known literature describing the use of NVR in communities and schools (Omer, 2004; 2011). To this literature, we would like to contribute how our team have drawn on systemic concepts in our delivery of NVR in schools.

One of the reasons for such a connection is the professional background of the main NVR co-ordinator. As a family therapist, she was trained in NVR back in 2009 by Elisabeth Heismann and Liz Day, the senior family therapists responsible for the development of NVR programmes in Oxleas NHS Foundation Trust. The facilitator team she developed joins up different ways of thinking, which is systemic in itself, and also continues to be systemically positioned.

NVR is understood by us as a social discourse; a 'system of statements, practices, and institutional structures that share common values. A discourse includes both linguistic and non-linguistic aspects; it is the medium that provides the words and ideas for thought and speech, as well as the cultural practices involving related concepts and behaviours' (Hare-Mustin, 1994, p19). In our school work, we have been developing language and practices that we hope will cultivate the discourse of non-violent resistance. When we started working with schools, we began by introducing new practices in parent-child relationships via NVR multifamily programmes, and have been following it up with exposing school staff to NVR language, concepts and behaviours.

In the spirit of postmodern thinking, we see our knowledge of NVR and its application to family and school contexts as multiple, fragmentary, context-dependent and local (Foucault, 1980), and we therefore tailor the approach to the needs of an individual family or specific school.

The obvious connection between systemic therapy and an NVR approach lies in the significance of repetitive sequences of interactions in maintaining difficulties (Burnham, 1986). Burnham recognised that these repetitive patterns, infused by sets of beliefs passed through generations and reinforced by emotions, are interconnected with systems outside of the family such as schools. Both systemic family therapy and NVR define an undesirable behaviour displayed by an individual not as a problem within the person but within the relationships in which the behaviour occurs. Omer (2004, p1-2) talks about how parent-child relationships can 'get caught in a vicious cycle', whereby reactions on both sides contribute to an intensifying pattern of escalation, and Burnham (1986, p10) similarly focuses on 'describing human dilemmas in terms of … an interactional description [which] encapsulates the pattern of relationships'. As Burnham (1986, p10) goes onto define, 'the basic unit of analysis, description and intervention must become the relationship'.

In NVR, this pivotal concept is expressed by a slogan: 'connection before correction'. It refers to an observation that in order for a child to be able to accept parental authority, there needs to be reciprocity (Burnham, 1986). One of the ultimate goals of an NVR intervention is the repairing of relationships previously characterised by symmetrical (hitting back, 'I'm the boss – no I am') or complementary (giving in) patterns of escalations by shifting it to reciprocal connectedness (Omer, 2004).

The systemic concepts behind such work may also be linked with Co-ordinated Management of Meaning (CMM). Most relevant to the NVR work we do is a question posed by Cronen and Pearce, the proponents of this theory: 'what part do we play in shaping the choices of others?' (Oliver, 1996, p247).

In our pursuit of stopping violence and/or self-destructive behaviours, we become curious about certain stories that are clung on to persistently, and the underpinning beliefs that need to be challenged to loosen the grip of these narratives. During our work we have heard stories of children being unable to control their actions or being spiteful by nature; that a school's response to students is not to be challenged; or that the parent is solely responsible for the child's outcomes.

According to CMM (Pearce, 1994) there are two sides of human experience, stories told and stories lived. The stories told are an aspect of us when we tell stories about us and the world in terms of our hopes, aspirations, dreams. The stories lived are concerned with the physical world when we attempt to put those stories told into practice on daily basis.

NVR allows a transformation. In systemic terms, the transformation of the stories told into stories lived involves using hypothesising, curiosity and circularity proposed by the Milan Associates (Cecchin, 1987). Therapists are urged to 'give up the attempt to direct people' (p 408) and avoid an illusion of control in a similar fashion to which, in NVR, we explore with participants, 'who we really have control over – clearly not over the children…'. Unwillingly, parents or school staff accept that they can only control themselves. An encouraging number of participants speak about this realisation, reporting that the control over their own responses gives a sense of empowerment and dignity. In CMM terms, a child whose parents and teachers no longer feel helpless and hopeless in the face of the problem is also left with different choices of response.

> *'Think positive. It's not about changing your child's behaviour… It's about changing how you cope with the behaviour. It's about taking care of how you feel.'* Parent facilitator

CMM helps to map out a repetitive pattern of communication that the majority of participants experience, as a 'charmed loop' (Pearce & Cronen, 1999; Oliver, 1996). **Figure 19.1** sets out the familiar vicious cycle of repetitive

## Figure 19.1: The escalation cycle

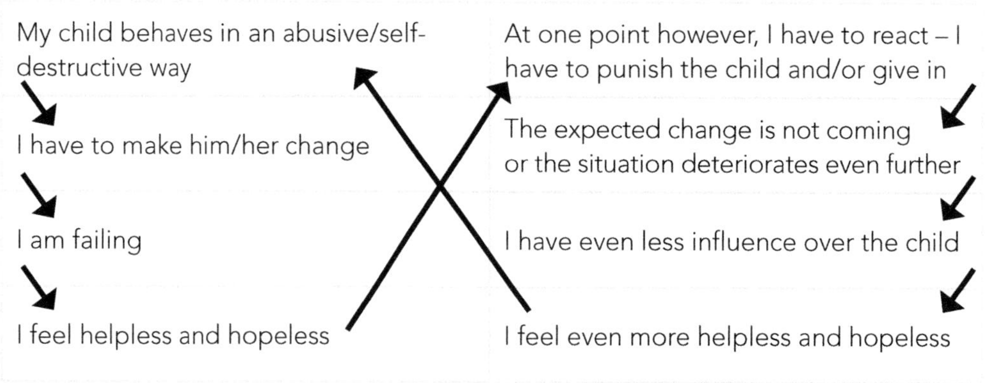


 

Such a loop is presented to participants in a kinaesthetic way when one travels on an imaginary line between one statement and the other only to come back to the first one. It becomes clear to participants that it is a vicious cycle, which if not interrupted will lead nowhere at best, or to a total breakdown of the relationship. Michael White (2007) describes that if a relationship with the problem becomes more clearly defined, a range of possibilities become available to revise this relationship (p26). In our programme we found that exploring this communication dance increases participants' curiosity and motivation to find out for themselves how NVR can help to break the pattern.

## Figure 19.2: Non-violent resistance

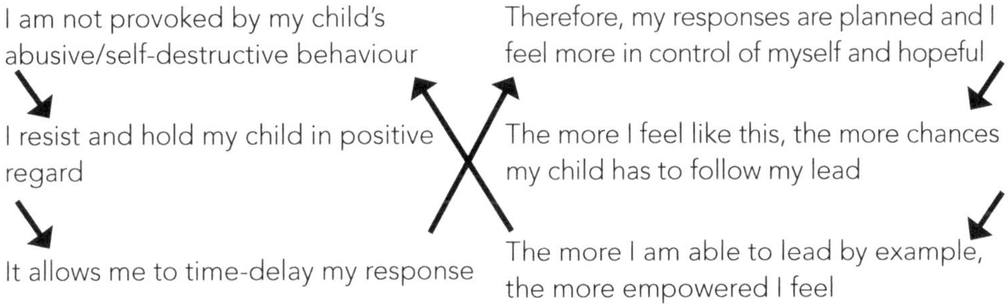


Lastly, we remain very mindful of aspects of power within our work. In family therapy we recognise that unacknowledged power struggles within therapeutic relationships are detrimental to the therapy. Working within schools, there are often power imbalances between parents and school staff; parents seem to be in a very vulnerable position in relation to teachers, and teachers' vulnerabilities are very often not acknowledged. Things can therefore become a 'blame game' in which schools blame parents for children's destructive behaviours and vice versa. NVR allows a re-frame such that we are not fighting against, but rather for, the child.

The inclusion of parent facilitators is also a crucial disruption to the power imbalance between participants and facilitators. They are more likely to be from the same social and cultural system as participants, and also to have experienced the disempowerment of their children's destructive behaviours, and the systemic responses this can elicit from schools, social workers and healthcare professionals.

# Description of the practice

> *'NVR group work is very rewarding and helpful with your children, especially teenagers. It has given me a look from another side of giving your teenagers some control and trying to work out things together, even if it takes time. The bottom line is connecting.'* Parent programme participant

> *'I've learnt how to talk to my kids instead of shouting when they argue. I thank NVR for giving me different techniques to deal with the situation.'* Parent programme participant

The programme is done in three stages, each of them equally important.

## Pre-group phase

At this stage the facilitators' team of school staff, CAMHS workers and parent facilitators, who have previously been through the programme, is formed. An important purpose of these meetings is to create a team building experience where the facilitators can gain an understanding of each other's strengths, needs and preferences in relation to their role as NVR facilitators.

The first team action is to prepare publicity materials, the second is to run a taster session that allows candidates to break the ice with each other and the facilitators, and hear the 'testimonies' of parent facilitators who have been through NVR. We have well-practised techniques that convey some of the key concepts in concrete and interactive ways, for example the use of physical baskets to illustrate prioritisation of behaviours, and a role-play with a scarf and an iron to demonstrate connection before correction. Some parents have found this visual representation very emotionally affecting, to see how the relationship can be damaged or 'dropped', and ultimately reinforces their wish to keep holding the scarf.

The taster session is followed by individual interviews with participants, which include the referrer, the CAMHS facilitator and a parent facilitator. These aid engagement on a more personal level, and give parent participants the opportunity to connect with the stories of those who have been through the group, as well as make them feel more comfortable with the CAMHS facilitator in the presence of an already trusted professional, the referrer. During these meetings, pre-group outcome measures are taken and the participants' goals for doing the programme are discussed.

 

## Group phase

We followed the basic multi-family NVR programme (Day & Heismann, 2010). The main well-known NVR concepts were covered over the ten-week programme (Omair, 2004; 2011; Weinblatt & Omer, 2008; Jacob, 2011).

Each of the ten sessions is preceded where possible by a 30-minute facilitators' pre-session, during which the programme for the given session is revised. After each session there is a debrief in which any issues arising during the session are discussed. During that time a plan for the next session is made, tasks are allocated to each facilitator and actions are decided.

There are also NVR consultations/supervision for the team with a CAMHS NVR practitioner.

## Post-group phase

The NVR programme includes support after the completion of the group sessions. In the first instance the participants are invited to the NVR community of participants and practitioners. We also discuss with participants volunteering options – some would like to help with a next group, some would like to become parent facilitator trainees.

'Regular Parent Club' meetings are run by volunteers. Newly graduated participants are invited to attend the clubs that serve as a forum for NVR graduate parents to meet and exchange ideas, share difficulties, ask for support and meet up with like-minded people.

# Learning points

The main learning points from our experience of running NVR groups in schools are now presented with illustrating examples. A reference point for our observations and insights comes from comparing NVR groups run within CAMHS for parents of children who are in treatment, to NVR school groups.

## Joining

> *'NVR … can have an impact, from one teacher or school wide, depending on how it is developed, adapted and most of all consistently carried out. For NVR to have the biggest impact in schools and learning environments, schools must train their staff informatively and all staff must buy into its*

*techniques. The latter can be a huge challenge as lack of consistency from staff can be one of the biggest challenges in any school.'*
Head of year at a secondary school

A key difference between schools and mental health settings is the significance of warming up the context for NVR among school senior leadership, teachers and pastoral staff; what a systemic family therapist would call 'joining the grammar' of the organisational culture (Cronen, 2001, p26). We have learned to pay careful attention to the initial creation and strengthening of connections with key staff members in order to gain their interest in NVR.

A warming up process helps, for instance, to receive suitable referrals to the group. Good connections between a referrers and referred parents support the development of good connections between the referred families and facilitators. A parallel process seems to continue because over the course of the programme, many parents are then able to re-gain connection with their children. Both in systemic family therapy and NVR practice we must be mindful of consistency between the content of the programme and the process of delivering it, utilising the core concepts at every juncture. In the following example, setting up a supporter's network is essential to the whole process.

### From our practice

In one of the schools, the growth of NVR started within a relationship with a dear colleague, school counsellor and an NVR facilitator. In our consultations with senior staff we 'head hunted' those staff members whose mindset was convergent with NVR concepts. We worked on nurturing those relationships and ensured those staff members were offered NVR training offered by CAMHS.

Alongside this, we gave a presentation to all teachers raising their awareness of NVR. It was welcomed with interest as the message was delivered by a member of staff who participated in the parent NVR group and adapted NVR to her teaching and relationships with pupils, and was therefore someone from 'the inside'. Two impressive parent facilitators also shared their stories, which offered an insight into the child and parents' world. Professional CAMHS facilitators contributed to the session, strengthening a sense of co-operation between school and mental health services.

 

This led then to conversations with a head teacher and senior leadership staff about how NVR could be used as a whole school approach to behaviour and teaching. We all agreed that taking time and working from the grass-root level up would be the most sustainable approach. It was suggested that a school working group would meet with the CAMHS link worker to discuss details, inviting NVR practitioners whose experience and work was relevant to schools. Their expertise and conviction of the NVR approach introduced excitement into the working group whose members decided to study NVR principals and experiment with using techniques in their lessons and reporting back their insights. The NVR team supported them in their endeavour.

A second example came from within a faith school, where we worked hard to involve the school chaplain in the running of groups. We used the chapel as a venue. The NVR principals were translated into Christian values and the NVR practices and messages were validated by the chaplain. Parents therefore found NVR congruent with the school ethos.

To make sure that NVR is supported by other staff members, we offered mini presentations to teachers. Close links with learning mentors were maintained so that NVR was kept in mind and appropriate families were referred to the groups. In this school we involved teachers as supporters, effectively training them in some aspects of NVR by default.

## Multiple relationships

**Unlike in the CAMHS NVR group where there is a loose connection between referrers and group facilitators and participants, a school environment is a close-knit setting. It seems that all people involved in the NVR group are at least in dual relationships.**

### From our practice

Let's consider the example of a parent facilitator who was initially referred by the school to her first group as a participant. She developed a relationship with the group co-ordinator/CAMHS link worker, and had a pre-existing relationship with the school staff member who referred her. In her next group she played the role of a graduate parent supporting the co-ordinator in running the group, so this relationship shifts to a different level.

She is also the parent of a child attending the school. When she becomes a parent facilitator, her relationship with school staff changes because she is now co-facilitating NVR training for them. Her interactions with teachers went through a transformation which had not been experienced earlier by either her or the school staff.

Now consider a situation in which this parent's son got into trouble in school. A potential to publicly blame the parent for failing to 'NVR' her own son may elicit shame, and impact on her confidence in interacting with NVR group facilitators – 'Do I have a right to be called NVR facilitator?' Furthermore, it also impacts the parent-school partnership.

Such a situation happened in one school group, and thanks to the parent facilitator's conscious use of NVR in managing the incident involving her son, and the school staff's willingness to maintain a good relationship with the parent, the outcome increased the connection between the parent and school. Potentially, however, the relationship could have been broken.

In addition, parent facilitators meet other parents in each group, possibly parents of their child's peers. Interpersonal relationships within groups introduce another layer of complexity to the mix. The group co-ordinator also has to maintain a relationship with the referrers, who are essentially her seniors, often high in the school hierarchy, while also connecting to participants who may be in conflict with these school staff.

The link worker must also be involved in managing the long-term working relationship between the school and CAMHS as a service provider, as changes in this partnership will inevitably affect the NVR work on the ground. Any difficulties are best dealt with by using the NVR approach, methods and tools.

## Length of relationships

All the complexity of multiple relationships within NVR groups in schools is multiplied by the long span of those relationships. An ending of the NVR group does not end the on-going relationships parents and children have with school staff or the link worker has with all involved.

This is in a stark contrast with CAMHS groups, where facilitators have no more involvement with participants unless they join the next group as graduate parents or parent facilitator trainees.

 

Conversely, a school system can also seem incoherent and unpredictable. If staff turn-over is fast, it means that those relationships that were a base for interventions one term may not be there the next. Changes in whole school strategies may shift together with new leadership appointments.

It is therefore particularly important to have a forum to think regularly about issues coming up in relation to participants, their children and staff, and their mutual relationships, including the professional facilitators relationships with all the aforementioned. Regular pre- and post-group meetings, supervision and briefings with senior leadership involved with NVR implementation maintains the connection with members of the NVR community and utilises support networks.

## Facilitating support and vulnerability in an unsafe environment

> *'In my role in a Pastoral setting … I often have conversations with parents who are beside themselves and don't know what to do or where to turn when their young person may be presenting or displaying challenging behaviour within the home and in school. This can often leave parents feeling unable to cope. Parents can often feel overwhelmed and unsupported and may at times present as being defensive. NVR keeps me interested as it is a tool used to support parents to effectively rebuild their relationships with their child. It enables the parent to think in a different way about what the issue presenting can be and also gives them different strategies to use. The results can be seen in school when the parents engage as they feel equipped to deal with the issues at hand. This then trickles down to the young person. It eventually helps the young person in school.'*
> Pastoral support worker in a secondary school

Again, in contrast to CAMHS, which is often associated with help and support, schools are often seen by referred parents as punitive and hostile. Shame and embarrassment are reported by participants as emotional responses to the school's suggestion that they do an NVR programme.

Cultural, ethnic and class differences often aggravate the strong emotional responses of parents, making the school an even less conducive environment for parents to make positive changes in their relationships with troubled children. It seems universally agreed that for an emotional change to happen, people need to feel safe in order to become vulnerable. Peter Jacob (2018) speaks about the need for a recovery environment in order to stimulate the participants' resourcefulness and their ability to rebuild relationships. To achieve those outcomes the above struggle is acknowledged from the very beginning with future candidates in tester sessions. Parent facilitators in their testimonies talk about their emotional journey and make a point of reassuring future participants that their current relationship with the school is transformed into one which is mutually respectful and supportive. The co-ordinator's job is to explore the power imbalance and painful feelings of shame and anxiety experienced by referred parents with school staff. It supports a shift in teachers' often habitual patterns of perceiving the situation, and invites them to get in touch with their own vulnerabilities.

A school can be shifted into becoming a genuine ally to parents, a place where parents can fully acknowledge their desperation and know that the school will alongside them to improve the situation. They can drop their defences and the school can activate their support systems. As Jakob (2018, p26) describes, it filters into the home environment, 'transforming relationships within the larger system to facilitate an emotionally stable environment'.

In one school setting, we found supporters a particularly important NVR principle to emphasise, and one which could be enacted with immediate effect due to the groups being run within the school. A mother and father who had felt isolated with shame for some time due to their son's violence were enabled to speak with a learning mentor immediately after one session to plan an announcement to be conducted at school. As well as breaking the silence about their child's behaviour, supporters established within the school via the NVR programme were able to reinforce the messages received at home about non-negotiable behaviours.

## Recruitment via 'recommendation'

In CAMHS groups, participants are referred by clinicians with whom they have mostly positive and strong relationships. In some ways, the referrers serve as a secure base during the period when participants form their relationships within the group. In schools, parents' relationships with school staff is not therapeutic and is therefore neither deep nor strong. For a referred parent to accept the referral and engage with the programme a robust recruitment process needs to take place.

We realised that the chances for engaging candidates are highest when the referrer, referred, professional facilitator and a parent facilitator have a chance to meet to discuss any difficulties and explore how NVR could be useful in improving the situation. In NVR terms, this process favours a relationship as grounds for future behavioural change – connection before correction.

 

## Conclusions

> *'NVR can and does work in schools as it focuses on building families' relationships often helping parents regain parental presence. This can then mean that the parent and young person have a more positive experience within school and with school staff. I hope to see NVR continuing in schools as it is important for work to be done in this way, as it can trouble shoot the root cause of an underlying issue by working with parents directly. It can be an extremely effective tool and a strong link between home, school and CAMHS. It also enables the school to maybe work in a different way or have a different approach with the young person and family.'*
> Pastoral manager in a secondary school

Introducing NVR in schools has been an invaluable learning curve, and we hope that the learning points have illustrated some of the hard-won insights:

- It is necessary to **join** the culture of the school and understand the system from the inside.
- Establishing NVR in schools involves being in complex and changing **multiple relationships** and positions in relation to staff and parents, and them in relation to each other.
- These **relationships** may be **of considerable length**, given that children hopefully remain in an educational setting for at least five years, and parent facilitators may be part of a system even longer than this.
- It is important to be mindful that **support and vulnerability are being facilitated in an (often perceived) unsafe environment**.
- The bonds of attachment in existing relationships can be drawn on in regard to **recruitment via recommendation**.

Undeniably, our actions are intertwined within the context in which they occur. We would therefore like to encourage readers to ask how this account could be tailored to your specific context, rather than simply asking how you could replicate this system of working.

The process described is clearly a challenge for those who wish to embark on it, however they need not be put off by the complexity of school cultures. A progressive approach to embedding NVR within a school's ethos is possible, introducing it at different depths, or starting with a single member of staff whose perspective seems to align most closely.

True to NVR history, we see the potential of connecting families with each other to share stories and expertise at a grass-roots level, and transforming how relationships between parents and schools are structured, enabling second-order change and bringing schools into the heart of local communities.

## Appendix: an introduction of the main concepts – connection before correction

As in mini-presentations to school staff, further physical props of an iron and a scarf are used in a roleplay to introduce the core concept of 'connection before correction':

'Please look at this scarf. It represents a bond between a parent and child, who hold it at opposite ends. The scarf may be twisted, creased or artfully arranged, but its essence is connection. It keeps people together.
At times, one person may drop the scarf, and a child finds themselves detached. Now they may need to seek somebody else to hold the other end of the scarf, or find themselves grabbing another person's scarf because it looks more attractive or may be more robust. Being connected is very important to all of us.

The dropping of the scarf represents a difficult circumstance in the parent's life, which may impact the parental presence with the child, for example parental mental or physical illness, bereavement or a new relationship.

Causes of the child's disconnection might be related to outside home influences, such as the internet, or additional special needs that interfere with the way the child interacts with others (e.g. ASD).

NVR, in such instances, is used to pick up the scarf – to reconnect.

Perhaps the scarf stays securely in the parent's and child's hands but the fabric of it is battered and full of holes. Maybe the parent or child tries to iron the creases in the scarf with the iron too hot for the delicate fabric of their relationship? Might it be too harsh disciplining and too little nurturing? Too many escalations with too few reconciliation gestures?

The scarf, even if in good condition and held tightly, will be affected by a polluted environment. It may get stained by other people's spillages. Our relationships are not isolated from our contexts, and therefore the impact of the circumstances outside the home may be significant.

 

In such cases, NVR would be used to maintain the scarf in as good condition. Ironing creases are important – disciplining is necessary, yet the manner in which it is done makes a difference to the well-being of the relationship. Gathering and utilising a supportive network of people who are beneficial for the relationship would be another.

The question is, what is the scarf for? If it is held and the fabric is strong, using it to lead someone proves easy. If pulling the child back onto the right track or heavy tugging is necessary, both the parent and child need to be closely linked.
The principals and techniques of NVR are about 'connecting before correcting'. It is about finding effective ways of maintaining or repairing the relationship.
You lead and your child follows. Then your child leads, and you may find yourself willingly going where they want to take you.'

## References


Burnham J (1986) *Family Therapy: First steps towards a systemic approach*. London and New York: Routledge.

Cecchin G (1987) Hypothesising, Circularity and Neutrality Revisited: An Invitation to Curiosity. *Family Process* **26** (4).

Cronen VE (2001) Practical theory, practical art, and the pragmatic-systemic account of inquiry. *Communication Theory* **11** 14–35.

Day L & Heismann E (2010) *Non-violent Resistance Programme*. Brighton: Pavilion Publishing and Media.

Department for Education (2016) *Mental Health and Behaviour in Schools: Departmental advice for school staff* [online]. Available at: https://www.gov.uk/government/publications/mental-health-and-behaviour-in-schools--2 (accessed October 2018).

Foucault M (1980) *Power/Knowledge. Selected Interviews and Other Writings 1972-1977*. New York: Pantheon Books.

Hare-Mustin RT (1994) Discourses in the mirrored room: a postmodern analysis of therapy. *Family Process* **33** (1) 19–35.

Jacob P (2011) *Re-connecting Parents and Young People with Serious Behaviour Problems – Child-focused practice and reconciliation work in non-violent resistance therapy*. Tel Aviv: New Authority Network International.

Jacob P (2018) Multi-stressed families, child violence and the larger system: an adaptation of the nonviolent model. *Journal of Family Therapy* **40** (1) pp25–44.

Leppington R (1991) From constructivism to social constructionism and doing critical therapy. *Human Systems: The Journal of Systemic Consultation and Management* **2** pp79–103.

Omer H (2004) *Non-violent resistance. A new approach to violent and self-destructive children*. Cambridge University Press.

Omer H (2011) *The New Authority: Family, school, community*. Cambridge University Press.

Oliver C (1996) Systemic eloquence. *Human Systems: The Journal of Systemic Consultation and Management* **7** (4) pp247–264.

Pearce WB (1989) *Communication and the Human Condition*. Carbondale and Edwardsville: Southern Illinois University Press.

Pearce WB (1994) *Interpersonal Communication: Making social worlds*. New York: Harper Collins.

Pearce WB & Cronen VE (Version 1. August 1999; Revised January 2004). *Using CMM. The Coordinated Management of Meaning*. San Mateo California: A Pearce Associates Seminar.

Weinblatt U & Omer H (2008) Non-violent resistance: a treatment for parents of children with acute behavior problems. *Journal of Marital and Family Therapy* **34** pp75–92.

White M (2007) *Maps of Narrative Practice*. New York & London: W.W. Norton & Company.

 

# Chapter 20: New Authority in schools – the PEN programme

**By Idan Amiel and Tal Maimon**

## From NVR to a (New) Authority concept

In the year 2000, Professor Omer from Tel Aviv University published his first book on parenting: *Parental Presence: Reclaiming a leadership role in bringing up our children*. It is important to understand that our team's work back then focused on aggressive children's behaviours. Trying to figure out a unifying concept for parents as to how they might protect their children from violence and self-risk, we came across the philosophy of non-violent resistance (NVR). In our view, NVR is more than a theory, it is a state of mind, an attitude or a way of life, set out by Gandhi and Martin Luther King. NVR served not only as a compass in our work with parents, but in a way it also helped us to find our next working place – Schneider Children's Medical Center of Israel (SCMC).

SCMC is a comprehensive, highly specialised care hospital – the only one of its kind in Israel and in the Middle East. The hospital is dedicated exclusively to the well-being of children and adolescents and receives patients from the Palestinian Authority, from Jordan and other countries in the Middle East. The Cornerstone Scroll beneath the building's foundations states, 'This hospital, dedicated to the inherent right of every child to live a healthy life in a peaceful world, will stand as a "bridge to peace" linking this nation to its many neighbours'[9]. No other place could serve our team's purpose better – to create a change with NVR in a violent region like the Middle East, and that is where, in 2004, we founded The Parents' Counseling Clinic. The Parents' Counseling clinic is the only outpatient clinic at SCMC of which its sole 'patients' are parents. While the slogan of Schneider Children's Clinic is 'It's all about the child', our slogan at the parents' clinic is 'It's all about the parent'.

In the following years, the variety of difficulties confronting the parents that asked for our help at SCMC expanded dramatically, and in many cases were not

9 For more information, visit https://www.schneider.org.il/eng

 

connected to children's violence. Issues like anxiety, computer overuse, unsafe driving, school refusal etc. persuaded us that a broader framework for our work was needed. Preventive components such as vigilant care had to be added to our programme in order to help parents (Shachar-Lavi, 2011). But the most drastic change in our working concept was created when we started to implement NVR with teams in residential settings, psychiatric wards and schools.

Just like parents, we found in our work that teams in residential settings and schools feel helpless in the face of a variety of extreme children's behaviours (aggression as well as avoidance and anxiety). Our slogan at SCMC then changed again, from 'it's all about the parent' to 'It's all about the caregiver', and the concept of New Authority started to form.[10]

In this chapter we will focus on our work in schools, present some of the New Authority guiding principles for teachers, and present a case study to demonstrate those principles and ideas.

## (New) Authority and schools

The traditional figure of the authoritarian teacher – stern, pedagogical and disciplinarian – has largely vanished from modern classrooms in the Western world, and in today's social climate it is neither desirable nor possible to recapture the authority that teachers once held the past. In our view, Western culture is at a crossroads; the more liberal approach to education has proven unsatisfactory and only a partial answer to children's needs, while the more authoritarian approach of the past is no longer valid in a world characterised by greater transparency and a more critical relationship to authority. How, then, can teachers build the authority to influence our youth but in a way that is valid an acceptable in today's world? It is from this crossroads that we have developed the New Authority programme for schools.

this crossroads that we have developed the New Authority programme for schools. It is important to note here that, unlike the parental counselling at SCMC which is measured in weeks, the counselling in school settings is measured in spans of many months. Changing attitudes regarding authority in a multi-participant educational staff is more complex than changing the attitudes of two parents towards their authority at home. The work of our New Authority team is therefore more complicated and challenging in schools.

10 A full summary of this process is provided in Idan's introduction to the book, *The New Authority: Family, school and community* (Omer, 2011).

 

# The PEN programme for schools – fundamental principles

The key starting point in our work with parents is to recognise and understand the parents' distress rather than blame the parents for their children's behaviour. A similar recognition evolved in our work with teachers – we emphasise the overwhelming difficulties facing teachers today, and our PEN programme centres on developing in teachers an NVR state of mind to empower them. The acronym PEN reflects three significant dimensions in the New Authority concept: **P**resence, **E**mpowerment and **N**et of support.

**Presence –** Presence is the central motif in the construction of the New Authority. The programme emphasises the importance of the teacher's presence in the student's life, in the classroom and in the hallways and courtyards of the school.

**Empowerment –** Another critical message in our programme is the empowerment of educational figures in the school, and the gaining of authority. This stance is of great importance and teachers sense it right from the start of the programme. Counsellors often arrive at the schools with a basic attitude that says, 'we're here to help you perform better and improve the students' condition'. Our basic position is, 'we're here to help you improve *your* situation as teachers, and deal with the difficulties you face due to a variety of student's misbehaviours'. It is important to realise that this position is not a mere slogan. The rationale behind it is that our 'client' is the teacher/principal and not the students. The basic belief that guides us is that empowering parents and teachers will lead to an improvement in the condition of the students.

**Net of support –** The best metaphor to describe the difference between the old authority and the concept of the New Authority is *authority as a support net*, instead of a rigorously hierarchical pyramid. The power of the New Authority figure is measured in their ability to create as many connections as possible, with colleagues, with parents and with the community in which the school is located, which enables the weaving of a network that supports their actions. We assist teachers in this regard. From our perspective, the support network is a network of authority figures, and as such it doesn't need to include the students. The students, if they wish, can of course join (and most of them indeed do it later on) but it is important to understand that our '(new) authority net' is first and foremost a net of adults who take responsibility for resisting some of the students' behaviours.

# Some basic tools from the PEN programme

## The bookmark

There are quite a few methods that have been developed to illustrate to teachers how to deal with escalation processes during class. One of the favourites among our staff is 'the bookmark'. This de-escalation tool is simply a short sentence which the teacher addresses to the student during an argument or confrontation: *'We're both angry right now, we'll stop that, and we'll talk about it at the end of the lesson. I ask you to sit down and continue working.'*

We call this a bookmark because a bookmark has two main roles. The first is to close a book at a certain point – just as the teacher 'closes' the argument. The student might continue to argue but as long as the teacher doesn't respond, there is no argument; the teacher remains silent and still at this point. But the bookmark's second use is to re-open the book at the exact point later. The phrase, 'we'll talk about that at the end of the lesson' is designed for that purpose, and at the end of the lesson the teacher calls the student over. The reaction of the teacher at the end of the lesson is solely up to their discretion, but the important point is that they did not respond in the heat of the moment – they delayed their response. The reader who is well-versed in our approach has probably recognised that this is a simple and effective application of the famous slogan: 'Strike the iron while it's cold!'

The 'team bookmark' is a simple variation of the basic bookmark – under certain conditions, in response to escalating behaviour by a student, the teacher may respond with a short sentence: 'We don't accept this sort of behaviour at our school'. The teacher closes the argument but does not invite the student for discussion at the end of class. Instead they inform another teacher about the incident. That's why we call this a team bookmark – one teacher places the bookmark and other re-opens the incident later. The message, 'we', trickles down to students but mostly grows in strength among the teaching staff. The change from 'I' to 'we' is a significant milestone in the change of perception from a lone (old) authority to a (new) team authority.

It is important to understand that the isolation and loneliness of teachers is structured into their jobs – the teacher stands alone in a classroom most of the day – and this work environment also becomes a state of mind. A central condition to escaping this isolation is to begin thinking and reacting as a team: 'we' instead of 'I'. But acting as a team does not occur easily. Teachers must acquire personal experience of joint responses in order to internalise the stance of 'we'.

 

## Mutual support: the announcement and the sit-in

The announcement and sit-in are two powerful tools that allow teachers to demonstrate a peaceful, strong, cohesive and determined presence. The use of these tools is intended for cases where it appears that the situation in the classroom is not the consequence of the problematic behaviour of a limited number of children (which can be handled individually), but where violence and aggression have become the class norms. The announcement and a sit-in allow teachers to resist unwanted behaviours while addressing the class as a community.

### The announcement

The announcement is a statement of intent concerning the team's position and its plans for action. The announcement makes it clear to the class which behaviours the team is unwilling to accept. It represents a turning point, not only for the students but also for the teachers: from now on, everyone is committed to collaboration regarding the issues being announced. The meaning of the one-sided announcement is: from now on, staff members will act determinedly to put its content into action, despite probable attempts by students to continue their behaviours.

The announcement defines the unwanted behaviours in a clear and specific way. It is important to note that the announcement does not mean starting a war; alongside the clear resistance to specific behaviours, a message of care and concern for all students in the class should be stated. The announcement is written on paper and should be read in front of the class, with several educators also being present there. During the announcement, only one staff member talks, usually the classroom teacher, while the other adult participants in the announcement should support silently.

We recommend that the teacher uses a calm and decisive manner and avoids anything that might come across as threatening. Afterwards they hang the announcement on the wall, give a sign, and the whole team gets up and leaves the classroom.

After the announcement, we don't usually expect improvement of the specific behaviours mentioned, but from this moment on the teachers will start working collaboratively, with determination and perseverance against the behaviours defined in it. When a behaviour defined in the announcement re-occurs, each teacher will use the 'team bookmark' and it will serve for the next act – the sit-in.

### The 'sit-in'

The sit-in is used in response to the re-appearance of behaviours that were defined in the announcement, and their purpose is to convey to the class the team's determined decision to resist these behaviours.

During a sit-in the team enters the class at a time pre-determined by staff members, they close the door, and sit in front of the class silently on chairs that are brought in for this purpose. Only one staff member talks, and the rest support them silently. After everyone has sat down, the teacher who leads the sit-in describes examples of the behaviours that were 'team bookmarked' by the teachers since the announcement and asks the students to find ways to stop these behaviours. The leading teacher considers the solutions they come up with and decides if they are satisfying. If a proposal was positive and acceptable for the sit-in host, they gives the other teachers a sign to leave the classroom quietly, preceded by a positive statement that they will give the idea suggested an opportunity to work. If no solutions are brought up, the teachers wait for 15 minutes in silence. Before leaving, the leading teacher says, 'We still have not found a proper solution'.

It is important to keep in mind that the sit-in is not an act of retribution, but a statement. Do not think of it in terms of 'winning' or 'losing'. The initiative of the educational team, the surprise to the class, the duration of the stay in the classroom and the silence are the elements that pass on the message: 'We're determined to stop this behaviour'. The initiative, the silence and the determination are the aspects that rebuild the staff's authority through presence. It also needs to be understood that sit-ins are not about finding solutions. Students often change their behaviour without proposing any 'solutions'.

# The classroom as a community: a case study

## Background and sketching an intervention plan

The first step in our PEN programme is an assessment of a school's needs in a meeting with a steering committee. The steering committee includes two to three members from the school, with whom our training team is in constant contact and who leads the implementation in the school. The first meetings with the steering committee take place before the onset of the yearly programme and enable us to properly define the 'character' of the school and the emphasis required in our intervention. A school's character depends on many parameters, including the student's population, the staffroom dynamics, the level of parental involvement in the school, etc. Accurate assessments of school characteristics enable us to avoid pitfalls and correctly avail ourselves of the school's strengths and resources.

 

In one elementary school in which we were asked to implement the PEN programme, it was clear from the beginning that one of the sixth-grade classes should be our focus of intervention. Reports about students from this class stated that many of them were left unattended in the afternoon, were involved in smoking, thefts and violence. Over the past year, attempts to improve the situation failed mainly due to feelings of despair and fatigue among staff and the bad relationship between the parents and the team. Many families were single-parent families, who were busy with day-to-day survival and had no time to look after the children at home. The school's past attempts to involve them had so far encountered resistance, denial and defensiveness. Even in cases where there was willingness to co-operate with the school, the helplessness of the parents prevented progress.

The subject teachers reported that they were fed up and had no desire to go to the class. The homeroom teacher, who could better handle the class, reported that the subject teachers did not respond with the appropriate disciplinary measures, expecting her to take care of all the problems. She felt alone.

In the next meeting with the school's steering committee we briefly introduced the content and tools of NVR and the New Authority. We planned that the next meeting would be with all the subject teachers, and the next would be with the parents. The idea gradually formed for us that we would use announcements and sit-ins as actions that would resist the behaviour of the whole class. Our aim had three targets: to enhance the teachers' presence in the classroom, to increase the sense of partnership and mutual support among the teachers and help to build a constructive relationship with the parents.

## The meeting with the teachers and preparing the announcement

The first meeting with the teachers, which was planned as a three-hour workshop, was very charged, and so was the classroom teacher. She shared feelings of helplessness about the interference in her classroom and her sense of failure. She burst into tears when her fellow teachers shared similar feelings. Considering that about 15 students in this class were described as having very challenging behaviours and lacking any kind of parental supervision, this was not surprising.

Although it seemed at one point that the helplessness had become contagious among the teachers, the prepared plan with the steering committee helped to create concrete steps and gave everybody hope. Focus, clarity and cohesion were crucial at this point for the teachers. By focusing on the students' acts in the classroom, three behaviours were chosen to be on the announcement: physical and verbal violence against staff and other students, speaking without permission during class and walking around during lessons.

The teachers were instructed how to set a 'team bookmark' in case the behaviours declared at the announcement were repeated. After putting a team bookmark in place, the teachers were asked to return to their teaching as usual and record it in a class log. The teachers were encouraged to consult with one another about handling unwanted behaviours in accordance with the existing rules of the school, and the documented problematic behaviours were to be used in the next sit-in.

## Joining the parents

The next step was to bring in the parents and, despite the sceptical mindset of some teachers, who believed that this task would be almost impossible, the steering committee set a date for a meeting with the parents. The classroom teacher called all the parents personally in order to increase the attendance at the meeting. These private calls were time-consuming but made the forthcoming meeting a more 'special class event'.

Despite the initial worries of the teachers, the meeting went well. The steering committee members were able to overcome resistances by highlighting the goals that the parents and the teachers shared. Some parents agreed to become actively involved in the process of change, and a list of parents who were willing to come to the school during day time was made. Still, the parents did not know the exact plan at this stage, for example about the announcement and sit-ins, and were only asked if they could spare some time and join the teachers in their efforts. Transparency is an important pillar in NA, but in some cases when you lead the way, we have found it easier to reveal our plan step by step.

## Acting the announcement

One Tuesday morning, the participating teachers met in the staffroom, grabbed chairs and moved together to the classroom. The teachers entered the classroom, put their chairs in front of the students and sat down, without saying a word. The entry was a complete surprise to the students, who were totally shocked. Seeing the school director, the deputy, and most of their teachers entering one after the other created an impressive impact.

The classroom teacher who was the only one who stood waited a few seconds in silence and started to read the following announcement:

 

> Dear students of the sixth grade, we are gathered here, all teachers of this class and the school board, to express our resistance to the current state of the class. Henceforth, we will resist physical violence and verbal abuse against teachers and students. We will also resist walking around and talking without permission during class. We will do whatever it takes to stop these behaviours and involve others as necessary. We are not going to give in, nor give up on you as individual students and as a class! We will do whatever it takes to stop the verbal violence and disturbances in your classroom. It is our duty as teachers!
>
> Signed, your teachers and the school board.

The students, who were still shocked, listened quietly. When the classroom teacher finished reading she turned around to the announcement board and stapled the announcement to it. With a tense silence in the classroom, the sounds of the pins penetrating the board created an unexpected dramatic effect that symbolised the teachers' determination that change would take place. After a few seconds of silence, the classroom teacher gave a signal, and all the participating teachers left the room, without adding a word.

Afterwards, the classroom teacher, who had maintained a strong attitude throughout the announcement ritual, burst into tears saying: 'I don't feel alone anymore'. All the teachers supported her, expressing their appreciation for the way, she had handled the announcement and had represented all of them. A (new) authority state of mind and determination clearly started at this moment.

The parent's reactions to the announcement came immediately after. When one of the students told his mother about the 'strange' and dramatic entrance of the staff into the class, the mother told him that the parents already knew something was going to change and that they had had a meeting about it two days ago. The support net started to be woven… It was now time to involve the parents in a more direct and active way.

## The 'sit-ins'

NVR is a slow and gradual process, and support is a crucial element of it. The announcement only signified the beginning of change, but now support was needed. On the day after the announcement, those parents who had expressed their willingness to participate were called by the school counsellor (who was one of the steering committee members) and were invited to the first sit-in. A sit-in at school requires complex preparation (replacing teachers in classrooms, making sure parents can arrive at school during work hours etc.), so the first sit-in was scheduled in advance for the week after the announcement. The steering committee did not wait to see if the students would change their behaviour – even after a successful announcement our working assumption is that time, patience, presence, and several sit-ins are needed for the desired transformation to happen. During the week between the announcement and the first sit-in, the classroom teacher had gathered the documentation in the class log, which established the text that was to be used in the sit-in.

Two parents came to take part in the first sit-in. A few minutes before they joined the sit-in, they were instructed to keep silent and just support the team with their presence. When they entered the classroom, again the students were shocked, as it now became clear to them that the announcement was not a one-time event, and this time the staff team were supported by representatives of their parents.

While all the adults sat down in front of the class, the classroom teacher stood and began saying: 'We're all here, the school administration, teachers and your parents' representatives, because in the last week there were several problematic behaviours that we strongly oppose. Indeed, last week there were also positive behaviours in the classroom [she noted examples], but we are here because of the problematic behaviours, which we had announced as unacceptable' [here she noted detailed examples, referring to the day, time and class/break time in which they occurred].

At this point she sat down and said in a lower voice, 'We'll sit here together and wait for you to find a solution to those behaviours. What do you suggest?'

The classroom teacher wrote the suggested solutions on the class board and asked the class not to repeat solutions which had already been proposed. At the end of the sit-in, the classroom teacher announced, 'The staff will continue to oppose any sign of physical or verbal violence and disruption in the classroom. This is our commitment, and this is what we will do. We will not give in, and we will not give up on you. You are important and dear to us.' Everyone left the room except the class teacher, who stayed on to teach the class as if nothing had happened.

It is worth noting here, again, that the solutions suggested by the students are not the important part of a sit-in. After all, it's more about taking responsibility over your acts and not about creating a dialogue. NVR (especially the 'resisting' part of it) starts when dialogue ends, and the sit-in procedure is not about suggestions or dialogue, but about protest (in this case the adults protest against the students' behaviours). The most important aspect, from our point of view, was the teachers' strong experience acting together as a team, feeling potent and supported by the parents. New and strong ties in the net of support were woven during this act. A second sit-in was already scheduled for two weeks later, this time in the presence of even more parents.

## Together we stand, divided we fall

After the second sit-in, the steering committee gathered the staff to catch up on recent events and decide on the next steps. Teachers reported a significant change, almost dramatic, in class dynamics. It was clear that they felt they were no longer alone, they were struggling as a team and this change strengthened them significantly. The team effort also led to changes in the students. Almost all the teachers described an improvement in classroom atmosphere, which meant that for the first time it was possible to teach properly.

Only one teacher spoke differently. She almost apologised for being a 'party-pooper', but said that she did not feel any improvement in her class. It was important to emphasise that the difficulties that she was experiencing were not her private problem alone, but again something that should be approached by the entire staff. The NVR intervention in the class would need to continue, until there was a significant improvement for this teacher too. This teacher was chosen to lead the next sit-in instead of the previous teacher.

After four more sit-ins, the behavioural problems changed from being widespread to being sporadic, with just two or three students. The positive voices of the students began to get louder and the atmosphere totally changed. It was decided that NVR acts concerning the whole class should be stopped and individual treatment plans for two students were tailored.

It is worth noting that several months into the process, the paper on which the announcement was written was still hanging on the walls of the classroom. The students had endless opportunities, to rip it down, throw it away, or at least draw on it, but they did not.

# Concluding remarks

As we wrote at the opening of this chapter, our focus is not on the children but on adults. But when teachers and parents change their attitude and their state of mind, the students just follow. In our view NVR is about resisting children's behaviours, but in the end what all children need is to feel that a (new) authority is there, whether it is at home or at their class. The New Authority concept offers a perception of the school environment as a community, where all the authority figures work together, conveying to the children and young people in their care a message of presence and joint action: 'We are here, and we are not alone. We are together, and we are with you.'

The central focus of the PEN programme is to empower the authority of the educational staff at the school. Our central message to teachers is – we are here to empower you, and if you are not stronger and don't have more presence, we haven't done our job!

We believe that if we do not empower the teachers, and as long as the school staff do not feel sure of themselves and confident, it will be difficult to improve the students' state of mind.

To summarise the New Authority state of mind, we would define it like this:
The New Authority is about empowerment. Influential figures, like parents or teachers, need not be defined by their ability to control children but rather by their ability to **initiate**, whether it's initiating care, initiating support, and yes, in some cases, initiating resistance through NVR in order to build a safe community for our children.

The PEN programme defines tools and procedures for teachers and parents to act and feel empowered by their 'New Authority', and make it work best for the children in their care. We didn't write much about them and their feelings, but let's not forget that they are the main reason for using the New Authority intervention.

## References

Omer H. (2000) *Parental Presence: Reclaiming a leadership role in bringing up our children*. Phoenix Arizona: Zeig, Tucker & Co.

Shachar-Lavi I (2011) Vigilant care. In: F Van Holen, A Lampo & J Vanderfaeillie (Eds) *Applications and Illustrations of Nonviolent Resistance and New Authority in Family Therapy, Education and Psychiatric Care* (pp21–26). Brussels: VUBPRESS.

 

# A brief overview of NVR and glossary of terms

Concepts and interventions are explained here for the benefit of readers new to NVR. This is not an exhaustive list but covers terms that you may encounter in this book. NVR is a living practice and the NVR community is constantly evolving and changing and developing new practices. We like to think it is like an underground network of roots (called a rhizome), and you will find this metaphor used throughout the introduction.

Non-violent resistance is a form of political and social struggle in which people come together to resist oppression through their physical presence and embodied protest (e.g. occupations, sit-ins, marches and strikes). The concepts have been applied by Haim Omer and others to situations in which parents find themselves dealing with children who show extreme forms of violent, challenging, non-functional and (self-)destructive behaviour.

The most well-known exponents of political and social non-violent resistance are Mahatma Gandhi and Martin Luther King.

## Classic NVR ideas

- **Parental presence:** A child's or young person's sense that their parent is there for them, that the parent is a safe, solid and dependable person who can be relied upon. A child's sense that their parent knows their whereabouts and cares what they are doing. The child knows what their parent's values are and what they believe about right and wrong.
- **Rebuilding the relationship:** When relationships have become characterised by violence and coercion there are very few opportunities for people to relate more positively. The relationship needs to be rebuilt based on acknowledging the negative, escalatory patterns and committing to learn to adopt connecting ones.
- **De-escalation:** Parents learn to identify when things are escalating and to step out of the pattern. Two types of escalation tend to occur: one where the escalation ends in violence and another where the parent gives in. Parents often do both. Parents learn to wait until things are calm and respond instead of react, using the maxim 'strike when the iron is cold'.

- **Breaking the silence:** Parents tell others about the child's difficult behaviour and how they feel hopeless and helpless, and that they need help.
- **Supporters:** Parents identify individuals who can support them and their child; they are specific about how they want these people to help them resist the young person's challenging behaviours.
- **Reconciliation gestures (or 'relational gestures'):** Parents make regular small gestures of love and kindness towards their child. These are small gifts (items of food, repairs to things that have been broken, special messages, watching the child's favourite TV programme) that are made irrespective of how the child has behaved and without expecting anything in return or pointing out the act of kindness to the child. Reconciliation gestures are intended to help the parent enact feelings of warmth and love. If the gesture is spurned, parents do not react.
- **Active resistance:** Parents choose to resist attempts to engage them in escalation. They resist the temptation to have the last word. Or they begin to withdraw services and no longer respond to unreasonable demands (internet access throughout the night, bribing the child to attend school, unlimited 'taxi' and laundry services).
- **Announcement:** Parents carefully construct an announcement that they will make to their child explaining that they are going to resist the negative behaviour that they want changed in the family; that they love their child and they want things to be better. They commit to a non-violent stance (verbal and physical). There are no threats or warnings. The announcement is short and specific. Parents practise making the announcement until it embodies and resonates with both their love for their child and their stance of resistance.
- **Sit-in:** If the child repeats the behaviour/s that were addressed in the announcement (for example, punching a sibling), parents will plan a sit-in. They will enter the child's bedroom and sit down, announcing in a calm and quiet manner that they are going to wait there until the child can suggest a way of changing things. They offer to assist the child in thinking about ways forward. Then they sit quietly for up to an hour (depending on the age/ability of the child) to demonstrate their love and their commitment to working towards change in a peaceful way.
- **Helping siblings and others:** By taking time to listen to their experiences and explaining the changes in approach, parents support siblings and others who have been impacted by the child's destructive behaviours.

 

## Developments in NVR

The following is a collection of post-NVR ideas. These build upon the original NVR concepts by laying the foundations for alternative, evolving practices. Not everyone will use all, or even some, of the ideas listed here.

- **Three Baskets (Uri Weinblatt adapted from Ross Greene):** Parents prioritise unwanted behaviours by placing them in three differently sized baskets. The large basket contains the largest number of behaviours and is to be ignored; the medium-sized basket is for behaviours to negotiate over; and the small basket is for the one or two behaviours that the parent is going to resist actively. The small basket must not contain more than two things.
- **New Authority:** The new authority emphasises parents' self-control, and favours persistence instead of control of their child; taking mutual responsibility for escalations instead of blaming the child and holding them solely responsible for family break-down; choosing resistance instead of punishment, and transparency instead of secrecy. It is a new paradigm of authoritative parenting that promotes supervision, firmness and discipline, and replaces distance, power and hierarchy used in traditional authoritarian parenting. The metaphor of the parents' anchoring function for the child and the importance of social support become central components of a secure parent-child bond.
- **Vigilant care:** Vigilant care consists of three stages that can be compared to a traffic-light-system. The 'open attention' can be compared to the green light. Parents keep their eyes and ears open, stay vigilant for any warning signals during routine contacts with the child (school runs, meals). In the 'focused attention' (comparable to the amber traffic light), parents become more vigilant and talk to other people who are closely involved with the child (teachers, friends, grandparents). In the 'protective action' (comparable to the red light) parents and their supporters take action (announcement, sit-ins, active resistance, increased visual presence, protective actions). Parents regularly shift between these three positions.
- **The Four Core Parenting Values (Michael Grabbe):**

1. Safety of the child and of others.
2. Developing their full potential and abilities in order for them to have a good future.
3. Having good relationships.
4. Showing respect for themselves, their parents and others.

- **Graduate parent participation:** Parents who have completed an NVR programme become actively involved in all aspects of the NVR projects (groups, mentoring, presentations, writing, research) to share their experiences with new parents and others. They combine compassion, empathy, containment and support with the hope that others can overcome hopelessness and despair as well, which parents new to the approach can listen to and believe, and accepting more readily from them than from professionals
- **Fourth basket or rainbow basket (sometimes also called the flower basket):** The rainbow basket provides parents with the opportunity to re-connect with their unconditional love for their child by prompting them to recall special memories and forgotten qualities of the child. This enables the child to be viewed more holistically.
- **Loss of parental presence:** Parents are supported to acknowledge fluctuations in the levels of involvement and presence they have in their child's physical, emotional and social life, and how they relate to the development of unacceptable behaviours. By exploring their own experiences, unmet needs and developing an inter- and intra-personal awareness, parents affirm their parental values and become conscious how they communicate them. This enables them to (re-) build their parental presence.
- **Connection before correction:** This maxim does not mean making a connection *in order* to make a correction. It means *prioritising* connection with the child *over* correcting the child's behaviour. We have moved away from focusing on correcting or resisting behaviours towards a relational stance.
- **Connecting conversations (adapted from Uri Weinblatt's 'Recovering conversations'):** After the deconstruction of old patterns, parents can start developing new ways of being for and with their child and learn to *respond* rather than *react*. Once they are ready, they can rehearse with supporters some new ways of being with their child. Active responsive listening to the child, noticing and naming how the child feels, reflecting on their own or others' relevant experiences (without falling into lecturing and preaching), visualising or naming the child's unmet needs, putting themselves into their child's shoes and seeing things from their side, empathising and asking for forgiveness are all examples of reconnection. This is not an exhaustive or prescriptive list. Graduate parents' testimonies provide inspiration for new parents, who develop their own ways of applying the NVR principles.
- **Self-announcement:** Parents and carers look in a non-blaming and non-judgemental way at the painful feelings and experiences that stopped them from being effective in their parenting. They commit themselves to being present, aware and involved in changing their own part in the unhealthy

 

escalatory patterns acknowledging their own capacity and motivation for bringing about change.

- **Child's/Young Person's Announcement:** Announcements can also be made by young people to parents and carers when practitioners are working with them using NVR principles.
- **Looking after yourself:** Parents make time for themselves and for activities that they enjoy, restoring themselves and enhancing their capacity for giving to others.
- **Use of mindfulness in NVR:** Parents and carers learn different ways of mindfulness as a practice of clearing the mind of thoughts and judgements by being attentive to unconscious processes and bodily sensations, thereby helping them reduce thoughtless and reactive tendencies which usually evolve from and maintain patterns of conflict. Mindfulness helps parents to cultivate their parental presence by allowing them to relax and take care of themselves in a constructive way and to develop a non-judgemental and non-violent stance towards themselves and others.

* 9 7 8 1 9 1 2 7 5 5 0 8 0 *
BV - #0071 - 281025 - C0 - 246/186/14 - PB - 9781912755080 - Matt Lamination